Competency-Based Practicals in Community Medicine

As per Competency-Based Undergraduate Curriculum for the Indian Medical Graduate prescribed by Medical Council of India

Competency-Based
Practicals in
Community
Medicine

As per Competency-Based Undergraduate Curriculum for the
Indian Medical Graduate prescribed by Medical Council of India

Anjana Verma MD, DNB, MNAMS, DHFWM
Assistant Professor
Department of Community Medicine
Geetanjali Medical College and Hospital, Udaipur, Rajasthan

Jitendra Kr Meena MD, DNB, DHFWM, ACME
Assistant Professor
Department of Preventive Oncology
National Cancer Institute (NCI)
All India Institute of Medical Sciences (AIIMS), New Delhi

CBS

CBS Publishers & Distributors Pvt Ltd

New Delhi • Bengaluru • Chennai • Kochi • Kolkata • Lucknow • Mumbai
Hyderabad • Jharkhand • Nagpur • Patna • Pune • Uttarakhand

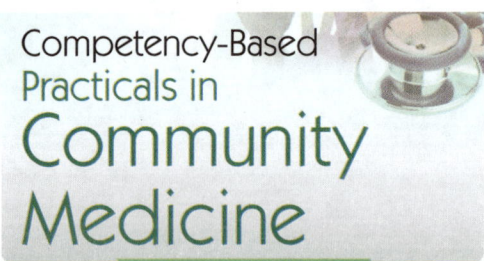

ISBN: 978-93-89261-82-0

Copyright © Authors and Publisher

First Edition: 2021
Reprint: 2022

Published by Satish Kumar Jain and produced by Varun Jain for
CBS Publishers and Distributors Pvt Ltd
4819/XI Prahlad Street, 24 Ansari Road, Daryaganj, New Delhi 110 002, India.
Ph: 011-23289259, 23266861, 23266867   Fax: 011-23243014
Website: www.cbspd.com   e-mail: delhi@cbspd.com; cbspubs@airtelmail.in.

Corporate Office: 204 FIE, Industrial Area, Patparganj, Delhi 110 092, India
Ph: 011-4934 4934   Fax: 011-4934 4935   e-mail: publishing@cbspd.com; publicity@cbspd.com

Branches

- **Bengaluru:** Seema House 2975, 17th Cross, K.R. Road, Banasankari 2nd Stage, Bengaluru 560 070, Karnataka, India
  Ph: +91-80-26771678/79   Fax: +91-80-26771680   e-mail: bangalore@cbspd.com
- **Chennai:** 7, Subbaraya Street, Shenoy Nagar, Chennai 600 030, Tamil Nadu, India.
  Ph: +91-44-26680620, 26681266   Fax: +91-44-42032115   e-mail: chennai@cbspd.com
- **Kochi:** 42/1325, 1326 Power House Road, Opposite KSEB, Kochi-682018, Kerala, India.
  Ph: +91-484-4059061-67   Fax: +91-484-4059065   e-mail: kochi@cbspd.com
- **Kolkata:** 147, Hind Ceramics Compound, 1st Floor, Nilgunj Road, Belghoria, Kolkata 700056, West Bengal, India
  Ph: +91-9096713055/7798394118, 9836841399   e-mail: kolkata@cbspd.com
- **Lucknow:** Basement, Khushuma Complex, 7 Meerabai Marg (Behind Jawahar Bhawan), Lucknow 226001, UP, India
  Ph: +91-522-40000032   e-mail: tiwari.lucknow@cbspd.com
- **Mumbai:** PWD Shed, Gala No. 25/26, Ramchandra Bhatt Marg, Next JJ Hospital Gate No. 2,
  Opp. Union Bank of India, Noorbaug, Mumbai-400009, Maharashtra, India
  Ph: +91-22-66661880/89   e-mail: mumbai@cbspd.com

Representatives

• **Hyderabad**	0-9885175004	• **Jharkhand**	0-9811541605	• **Nagpur**	0-9421945513
• **Patna**	0-9334159340	• **Pune**	0-9623451994	• **Uttarakhand**	0-9716462459

Printed at: Goyal Offset Works (P) Limited, Sonipat, Haryana, India.

Foreword

I am glad to know that the first edition of *Competency-Based Practicals in Community Medicine* is being released. This book is fully updated with the new curriculum implemented by the Medical Council of India (MCI) as per the international requirements of the World Federation for Medical Education (WFME). The content provided in the book is student-friendly, and is laid down in a precise and comprehensive manner. I congratulate the authors, Dr Anjana Verma and Dr Jitendra Kr Meena, who have done exemplary work. This book is highly recommended for undergraduate (UG) medical, dental, nursing, paramedical students and those preparing for postgraduate (PG) examinations. I am sure the students will benefit greatly from community medicine practical concepts detailed in the book.

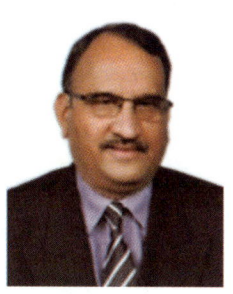

FS Mehta
Dean and Principal and Controller
Geetanjali Medical College and Hospital
Udaipur, Rajasthan

Preface

Over the years, there has been a widening gap between community needs and the availability of health care with traditional medical education approach. This has led the Medical Council of India (MCI) to devise and implement reforms in the medical education by introducing the Competency-Based Undergraduate Medical Curriculum (CBME). It focuses on learning pre-identified competencies for clinical practice and provides appropriate guidance for various teaching–learning methods and performance assessment. It aims to produce competent Indian Medical Graduates (IMGs) who can appropriately and effectively function as physicians of the first contact in the community.

This book has been designed as per the new CBME curriculum. All chapters have been formulated according to the specified competencies. The curriculum has been introduced in a concise but comprehensive manner to make it student-friendly whilst not deviating from fundamentals of community medicine practicals. This book will provide undergraduate (UG) and postgraduate (PG) students in medical and paramedical specialties a broad insight into the practical aspect of community medicine. We sincerely wish students and teachers will benefit immensely from the book and welcome their continuous feedback and suggestions for improvement.

We are very grateful to our respected teachers and seniors at the Department of Community Medicine, Maulana Azad Medical College, New Delhi, who inspired us to work hard. We are thankful to Dr FS Mehta, Dean, Dr. Mukul Dixit, Head, Department of Community Medicine and colleagues at Geetanjali Medical College and Hospital (GMCH) for their support and encouragement.

We sincerely thank Mr YN Arjuna (Senior Vice-President, Publishing, Editorial and Publicity) and the team at CBS Publishers and Distributors for taking up this project, beautifully designing and developing the First Edition of the book.

Anjana Verma
Jitendra Kr Meena

Contents

SECTION III
Epidemiological and Statistical Exercises

SECTION IV
Field Visits to Public Health Institutions

SECTION V
Additional Resources

Index of Competencies

SECTION II
Spots

SECTION III
Epidemiological and Statistical Exercises

SECTION IV
Field Visits to Public Health Institutions

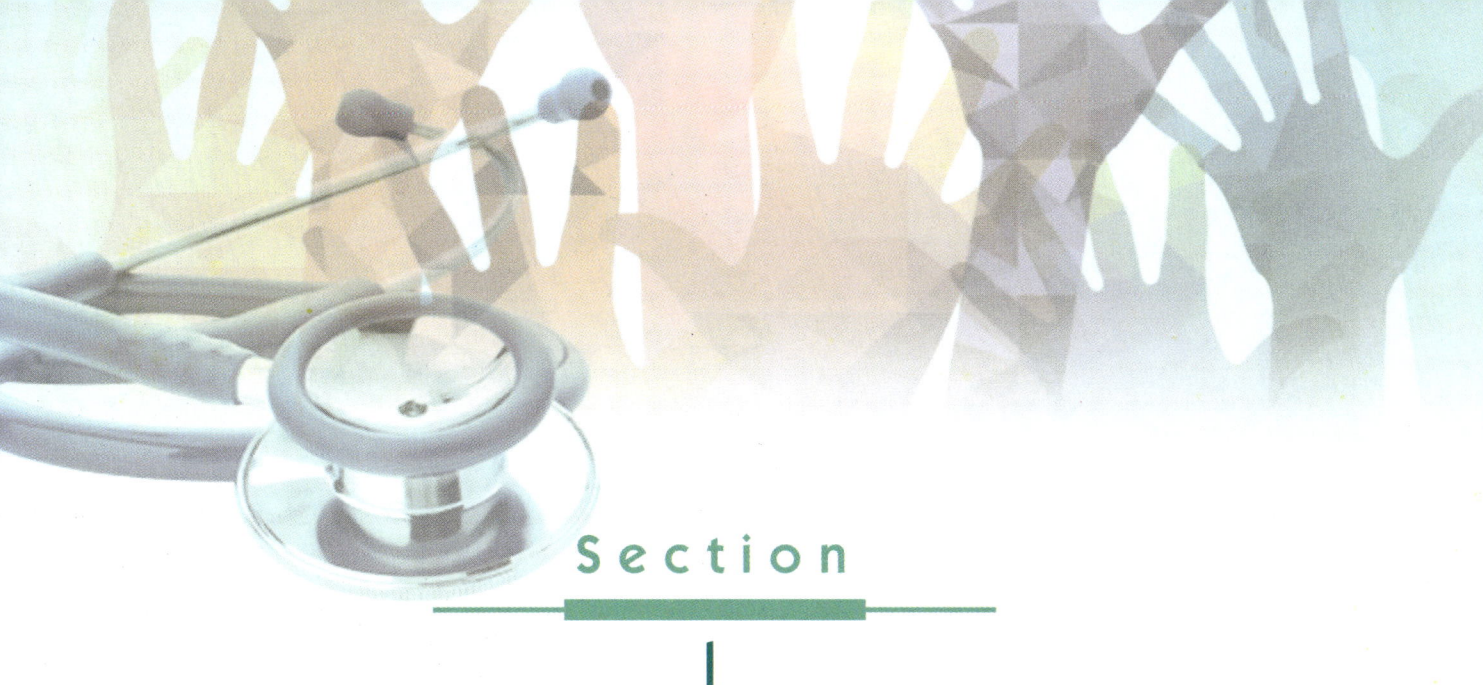

Section

I

Family Survey and Clinico Social Cases

- ◆ Spot Map of Field Practice Area

- ◆ Demographic Details and House Survey

- ◆ Immunization Status

- ◆ Personal Hygiene

- ◆ Environmental Health Status

- ◆ Socioeconomic Status

- ◆ Sociocultural Environment

- ◆ Preventive Check-up (ANC/ PNC, Under 5)

- ◆ Preventive Check-up (Other Individuals)

- ◆ Dietary Assessment

- ◆ Case Presentations (Diabetes, Hypertension, etc.)

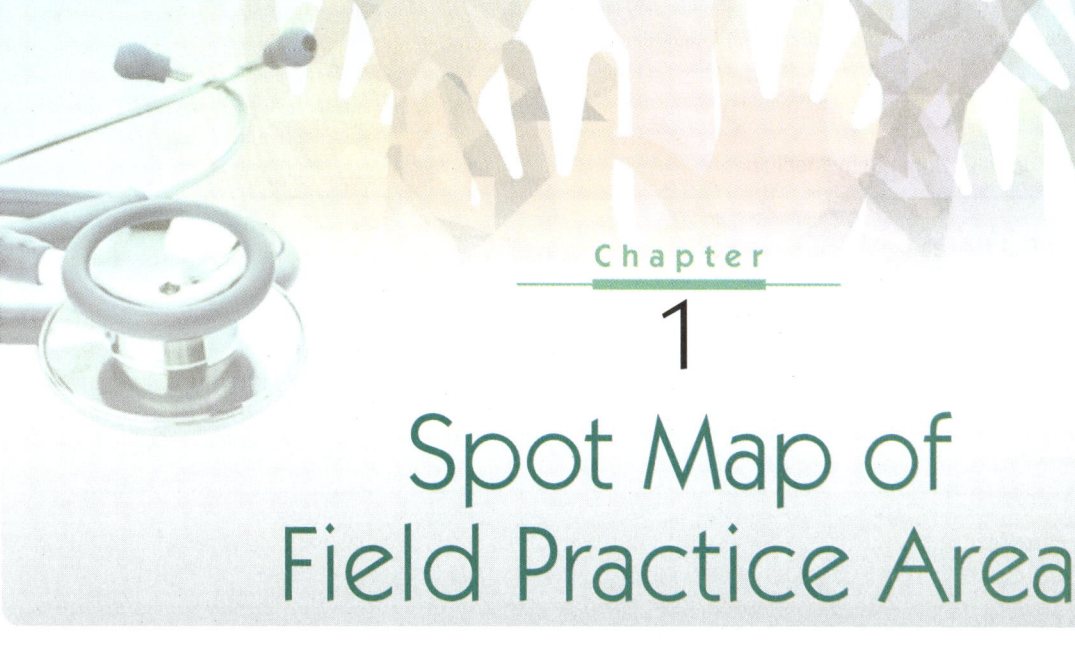

Spot Map of
Field Practice Area

Competency		Suggested teaching	Suggested assessment
CM2.1	Describe the steps and perform a clinical socio-cultural, and demographic assessment of the individual, family and community	Lecture, small group discussion, DOAP (Demonstration, Observation, Assistance and Performance) session	Written/viva voce/ skill assessment

Example of a Community Spot Map

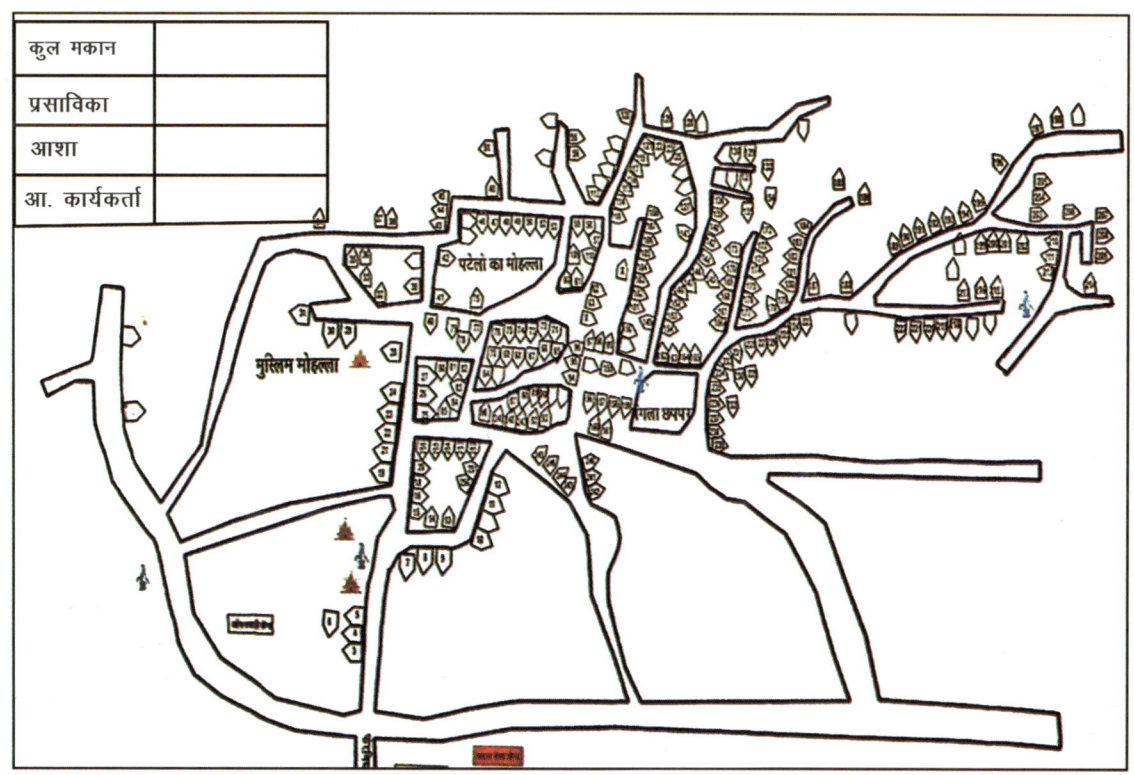

कुल मकान	
प्रसाविका	
आशा	
आ. कार्यकर्ता	

Demographic Details of Field Area

1. Name of the area ....

....

2. Age distribution ....

....

3. Sociocultural distribution...

....

4. Educational facilities...

....

5. Socioeconomic status ....

....

6. Health seeking behavior..

....

7. Other information ....

....

8. Total population ....

....

9. Gender distribution...

....

10. Principal mode of livelihood...

....

11. Literacy status..

....

12. Health/Anganwadi centres ....

....

13. Endemic diseases..

....

Demographic Details and House Survey

Competency		Suggested teaching	Suggested assessment
CM1.9	Demonstrate the role of effective communication skills in health in a simulated environment	DOAP sessions	Skill assessment
CM2.1	Describe the steps and perform a clinical sociocultural and demographic assessment of the individual, family and community	Lecture, small group discussion, DOAP session	Written/viva voce/skill assessment

A. Introduction

1. Respondent (name, age and gender):...

2. Address: ....

3. Setting: ☐ Rural   ☐ Urban (*Tick appropriate*)

B. Family Structure

1. Name of the head with the surname:...

2. Type of the family: ☐ Joint   ☐ Nuclear

3. Religion and caste: ☐ Hindu   ☐ Muslim   ☐ Others,   ☐ General   ☐ SC   ☐ ST   ☐ OBC

4. Annual income of the family:

   a. Per capita income:...

   b. Socioeconomic status: ☐ APL   ☐ BPL, Class: ....(*Chapter 6*)

   Total expenditure of the family:

   a. Food:..

   b. Medical:...

   c. Others (beedi/cigarette/alcohol/gutkha): ....

5. Profile of the family members:

S. No.	Name of family members	Relation to head of family	Age/ gender	Marital status	Education	Occupation	Income (per month)	Any disease
1.								
2.								
3.								
4.								
5.								
6.								

6. Nearest health care facility or provider: Name:………………….…………..□ Private   □ Government

7. Vital events in the family in the past 1 year:

   □ Births   □ Deaths   □ Marriage   □ Migration   □ Adoption   □ Divorce

8. Social security: □ Bank account   □ Ration card   □ RSBY   □ Ayushman Bharat   □ Others:………

C.   Environmental Conditions of the Family

1. House

a. Possession: □ Owned   □ Rented

b. Residing since................. (years)   □ Permanent   □ Temporary

c. Outset: □ Open   □ Closed

d. Construction of the house: □ Pucca   □ Kachha

e. Walls: □ Not plastered   □ Plastered-mud   □ Cement

f. Lighting: Natural: □ Adequate   □ Inadequate, Artificial   □ Adequate   □ Inadequate

g. Cross ventilation: □ Present   □ Absent

h. Overcrowding: □ Present   □ Absent

   If present, ...

   Criteria: □ People/Room   □ Area   □ Gender separation

i. Surroundings of the house:

   □ Open drains   □ Vector breeding sites   □ Waste disposal area   □ Stray animals

j. Domestic hazards: □ Present   □ Absent

2. Kitchen

a. Construction: ☐ Separate   ☐ Not separate

b. Fuel used for cooking: ☐ Smoke forming   ☐ Smokeless

   If smoke forming, smoke outlet: ☐ Present   ☐ Absent

c. Storage of general food items: ☐ Proper   ☐ Improper

d. Storage of raw food items: ☐ Covered   ☐ Not covered

3. Water

a. Source: ☐ Private   ☐ Public,   ☐ Piped   ☐ Borewell,   ☐ Others:…………………………………

b. Supply: ☐ Continuous   ☐ Intermittent

c. Storage of water: ☐ Open   ☐ Closed

d. Household purification of water: ☐ Absent   ☐ Boiling   ☐ Filtration   ☐ Others: ……………………

e. Fetching of drinking water from the container: ☐ Tap   ☐ Ladle   ☐ Dipping vessel

4. Sanitation

a. Sanitary latrine: ☐ Present   ☐ Absent

b. Location: ☐ Within the house   ☐ Attached to the dwelling unit   ☐ Away from house

c. Regularly used: ☐ Yes   ☐ No

d. Privacy consideration: ☐ Yes   ☐ No

e. Availability of water: ☐ Yes   ☐ No

f. Cleanliness: ☐ Satisfactory   ☐ Unsatisfactory

g. Floor: ☐ Slippery   ☐ Nonslippery

h. Solid waste disposal: ☐ Dustbin or covered container   ☐ Open

i. Frequency of collection and disposal: ☐ Daily   ☐ Alternate days   ☐ Irregular

j. Domestic animals in the house: ☐ Present   ☐ Absent

k. Rodents: ☐ Present   ☐ Absent

l. Arthropod Vectors: ☐ Present   ☐ Absent

D. Dietary Practices of the Family

a. Type of diet: ☐ Vegetarian   ☐ Non-vegetarian

b. Fruit/vegetable intake: ☐ Adequate   ☐ Inadequate

c. Calorie intake: ☐ Adequate   ☐ Inadequate

d. Protein intake: ☐ Adequate   ☐ Inadequate

e. Hand washing: ☐ Yes   ☐ No

f. Storage of cooked food: ☐ Proper   ☐ Improper

g. Prior cleaning of vegetables: ☐ Yes   ☐ No

h. Type of salt used: □ Iodized □ Not iodized

i. Type of oil used: □ Vanaspathi □ Sunflower oil □ Mustard oil □ Groundnut oil

  □ Others ....

E. Knowledge, Attitude and Practices (KAP) Regarding Health and Disease

a. How are diseases caused? □ Disease agents □ Diet-related □ Evil spirits/God □ Others
....

b. How are diseases treated? □ Medicine/surgery □ Holy intervention/God □ Others................

c. Preferred health care provider? □ Trained doctors (allopathic) □ Trained doctors (AYUSH)
  □ Quacks/faith healers

d. Proper age for marriage for girls? ....

e. The optimum number of children for a couple?...

f. Family planning: □ Desirable □ Undesirable.

g. How cholera is caused? ....

h. How malaria is caused? ....

i. How TB is caused? ....

j. What are the diseases transmitted by mosquito? ....

k. Enumerate some waterborne diseases:..

F. Summary

○ **Overall Family Health Assessment:** □ Excellent □ Good □ Average □ Poor □ Very poor

○ **Problems identified**

  ◆ |_____|

  ◆ |_____|

  ◆ |_____|

  ◆ |_____|

○ **Advise given/action taken:**

  ◆ |_____|

  ◆ |_____|

  ◆ |_____|

  ◆ |_____|

3

Immunization Status

Competency		Suggested teaching	Suggested assessment
CM1.9	Demonstrate the role of effective communication skills in health in a simulated environment	DOAP sessions	Skill assessment
CM1.10	Demonstrate the important aspects of the doctor–patient relationship in a simulated environment	DOAP sessions	Skill assessment

1. Immunization data (under five children):

Name	Age	Vaccines given								Status[#]
		At birth	6 wk	10 wk	14 wk	9 months	16–24 months	5 years	10 years	

[#] *Immunization status: Mark 'F' for fully immunized, 'P' for partially immunized and 'U' for unimmunized.*

2. Other vaccines *(Specify: Name of the individual immunized, vaccine and doses and dates)*

....

3. Vaccines not given by the due date

Name	Due vaccines dose not given	Reasons for delay/failure	Advice given/action taken

Personal Hygiene

Competency		Suggested teaching	Suggested assessment
CM1.9	Demonstrate the role of effective communication skills in health in a simulated environment	DOAP (Demonstration, Observation, Assistance and Performance) sessions	Skill assessment

4.1 Personal Hygiene Data

Personal hygiene	Parameters	1	2	3	4	5	6
Clothing	Clean/Dirty						
Hand wash with soap	Yes/No						
Body cleanliness	Yes/No						
Hair clean	Yes/No						
Eyes clean	Yes/No						
Oral hygiene	Good/Bad						
Ear hygiene	Good/Bad						
Skin disease	Clean/Dirty						
	Present/Absent						
Menstrual hygiene (if applicable)	Present/Absent						
Footwear use	Regular/Occasional/Never						
Associated health problems							

4.2 Overall Assessment

☐ Excellent   ☐ Good   ☐ Average   ☐ Poor   ☐ Very poor

○ **Problems identified**

- ◆ [   ]

- ◆ [   ]

- ◆ [   ]

- ◆ [   ]

○ **Advise given/action taken:**

- ◆ [   ]

- ◆ [   ]

- ◆ [   ]

- ◆ [   ]

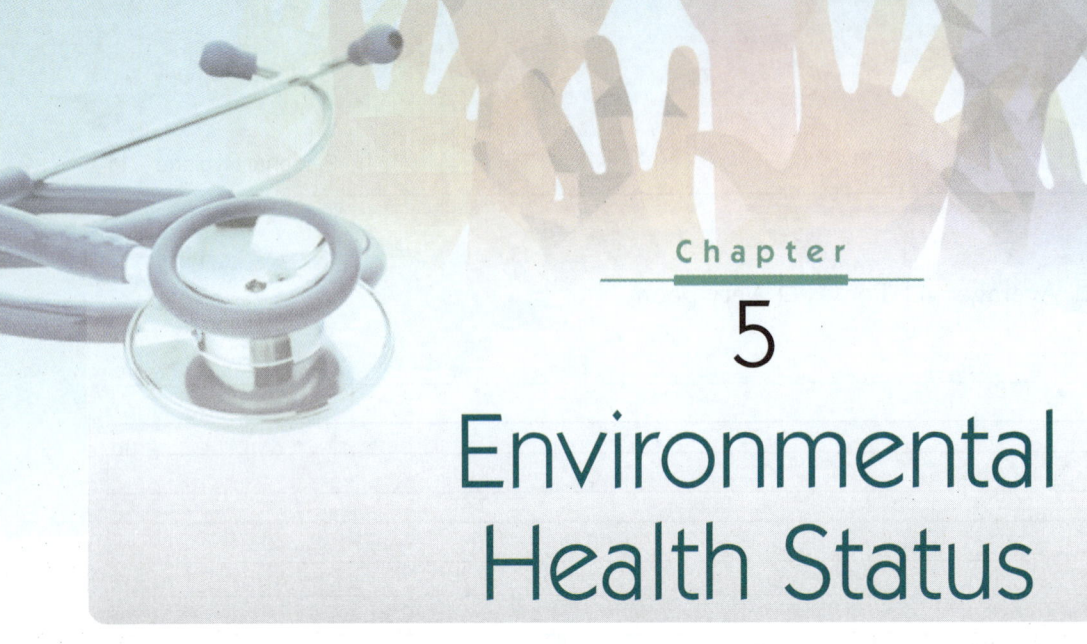

5

Environmental Health Status

Competency		Suggested teaching	Suggested assessment
CM1.9	Demonstrate the role of effective communication skills in health in a simulated environment	DOAP (Demonstration, Observation, Assistance and Performance) sessions	Skill assessment
CM3.5	Describe the standards of housing and the effect of housing on health	Lecture, small group discussion	Written/viva voce
IM25.13	Counsel the patient and family on prevention of various infections due to environmental issues	DOAP (Demonstration, Observation, Assistance, and Performance) sessions	Skill assessment

5.1 House Data

a. House.. ☐ Kutcha/☐ Pucca/☐ Semi-Pucca

b. No. of living rooms ....

c. Overcrowding: ☐ Present/☐ Absent

   If present,

   Criteria: ☐ People/Room   ☐ Area   ☐ Gender separation

d. Kitchen environment

   i. Clean/Unclean...

   ii. Separate: ☐ Yes/☐ No

   iii. Fuel used ....

   iv. Storage of food: ☐ Hygienic/☐ Unhygienic

e. Presence of pet animals (specify)...

f. Rats in the house: ☐ Yes/☐ No

g. Presence of arthropods in the house: ☐ Houseflies/☐ Mosquitoes/☐ Cockroaches/☐ Other

h. Sources of light:

   i. *Natural:*   ☐ Adequate /☐ Inadequate

   ii. *Artificial:*   ☐ Adequate/☐ Inadequate

5.2 Neighbourhood

House Surrounding

a. ☐ Clean/☐ Unclean

b. Locality :☐ Urban slum/☐ Resettlement colony/☐ Posh colony

5.3 Measurements of the House

Rooms measurement (in feet)		Ventilators		Windows			Doors		Ventilation
S.No.	Size (l × b × h)	No.	Size (l × b)	No.	Size (l × b)		No.	Size (l × b)	Satisfactory/ Not satisfactory

5.4 Water Supply

a. Source ....

b. Frequency: ☐ Continuous/☐ Intermittent

c. How drinking water is stored? ....

d. How water is taken out for consumption?...

e. Impression: ☐ Safe/☐ Unsafe

5.5 Excreta Disposal   ☐ Sanitary latrine/☐ Unsanitary latrine/☐ Open air

5.6 Waste

a. Is the family aware of environmental hazards of using plastic bags?   ☐ Yes/☐ No

b. Disposal: (a) Stored in   ☐ Open dustbin/☐ Covered dustbin

c. Disposed off: ☐ Daily/☐ Less frequently

   Mode of disposal ....

5.7 Surrounding of the House

a. Drainage: ☐ Open/☐ Covered

b. Garbage: ☐ Present/☐ Absent

c. Collection of water: ☐ Present/☐ Absent

d. Breeding of mosquitoes: ☐ Present/☐ Absent

5.8 Inspection for Breeding Places

a. Aedes mosquitoes: ☐ Not found/☐ Found (specify ....)

b. Anopheles mosquitoes: ☐ Not found/☐ Found (specify ....)

5.9 Overall Environment Assessment

☐ Excellent ☐ Good ☐ Average ☐ Poor ☐ Very Poor

○ **Problems identified**

    ◆ [   ]

    ◆ [   ]

    ◆ [   ]

    ◆ [   ]

○ **Advise given/action taken**

    ◆ [   ]

    ◆ [   ]

    ◆ [   ]

    ◆ [   ]

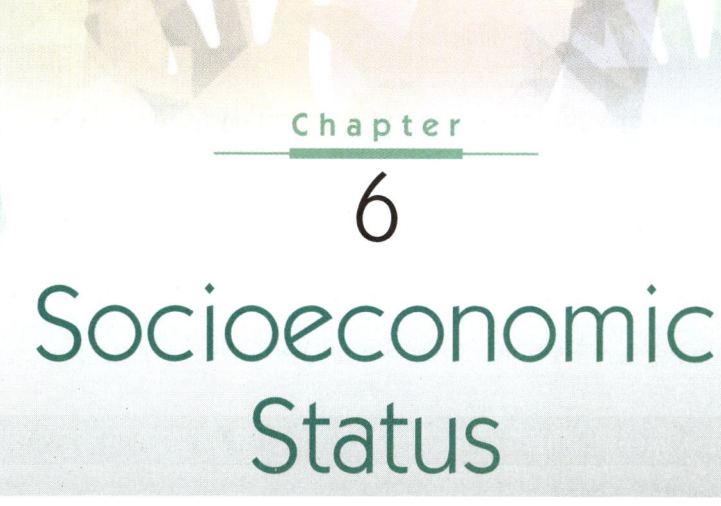

Chapter

6

Socioeconomic Status

Competency		Suggested teaching	Suggested assessment
CM1.9	Demonstrate the role of effective communication skills in health in a simulated environment	DOAP sessions	Skill assessment
CM2.2	Describe the correct assessment of socioeconomic status	Lecture, small group discussion, DOAP session	Written/viva voce/ skill assessment
CM2.5	Describe poverty and social security measures and its relationship to health and disease	Lecture, small group discussion	Written/viva voce

6.1 Income Source and Expenditure Pattern

1. Total monthly income (in rupees):..

2. Total monthly expenditure (in rupees): ....

3. Total monthly expenditure on food (in rupees):...

4. Total monthly health expenditure (in rupees): ....

5. Catastrophic health expenditure: ☐ Yes/ ☐ No
   (Catastrophic health expenditure defined as out-of-pocket payments on health in the recall period of 1 month equalling or exceeding 10% of total household expenditure)

6. Per capita income per month *(Total family income in a family divided by total family members)* ....

6.2 Socioeconomic Scales: Modified Kuppuswamy Scale (for Urban Area)

Occupation is classified as follows:

1. *Professional:* Lawyer, doctor, etc.

2. *Semi-professional:* High school teacher, lecturer, insurance inspector, musician, research assistant, etc.

3. *Clerical/shopowner:* Clerk, typist, junior accountant, elementary school teacher, shopkeeper, firm owner, station master, guard, news correspondent, salesman, insurance agent, etc.

4. *Skilled worker:* Mason, carpenter, mechanic, radio repairer, engine and car driver, telephone mechanic, etc.

5. *Semi-skilled worker:* Factory or workshop labour, lab and library attendant, car cleaner, petty shopkeeper, etc.

6. *Unskilled worker:* Porter, peon, watchman, domestic servant, etc.

Table 6.1:	Occupation of the head of the family	
S.No.	**Occupation of the head**	**Score**
1.	Legislators, senior officials and managers	10
2.	Professionals	9
3.	Technicians and associate professionals	8
4.	Clerks	7
5.	Skilled workers and shop and market sales workers	6
6.	Skilled agricultural and fishery workers	5
7.	Craft and related trade workers	4
8.	Plant and machine operators and assemblers	3
9.	Elementary occupation	2
10.	Unemployed	1

Table 6.2:	Education of the head of the family	
S.No.	**Education of the head**	**Score**
1.	Profession or honours	7
2.	Graduate	6
3.	Intermediate or diploma	5
4.	High school certificate	4
5.	Middle school certificate	6
6.	Primary school certificate	3
7.	Illiterate	2
8.	Plant and machine operators and assemblers	1

Table 6.3:	Total monthly income of the family	
S.No.	**Updated monthly family income in Rupees (2019)**	**Score**
1.	≥78063	12
2.	39033–78062	10
3.	29200–39032	6
4.	19516–29199	4
5.	11708–19515	3
6.	3908–11707	2
7.	≤3907	1

Table 6.4:	Kuppuswamy's socioeconomic status scale 2019	
S.No.	**Score**	**Socioeconomic class**
1.	26–29	Upper (I)
2.	16–25	Upper middle (II)
3.	11–15	Lower middle (III)
4.	5–10	Upper lower (IV)
5.	< 5	Lower (V)

BG Prasad Scale 2019 (for both Urban and Rural Areas)

Table 6.5:	Revision of the Prasad's social classification for the year 2019
Social class	**Revised for 2019 (in Rs./month)**
I.	7000 and above
II.	3504–7007
III.	2102–3503
IV.	1051–2101
V.	1050 and below

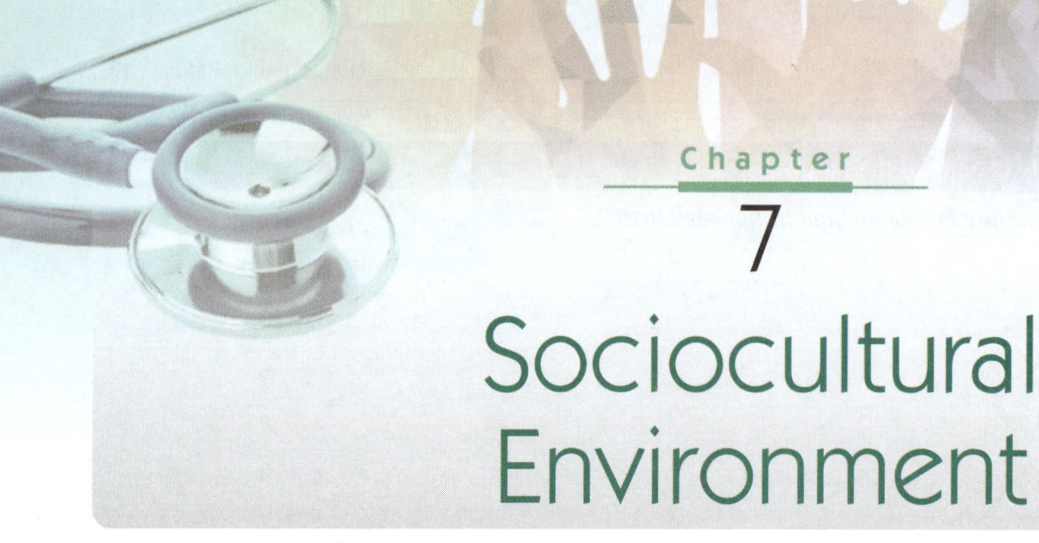

Sociocultural Environment

Competency		Suggested teaching	Suggested assessment
CM1.9	Demonstrate the role of effective communication skills in health in a simulated environment	DOAP (Demonstration, Observation, Assistance and Performance) sessions	Skill assessment
CM2.2	Describe the sociocultural factors, family (types), its role in health and disease and demonstrate in a simulated environment	Lecture, small group discussion, DOAP (Demonstration, Observation, Assistance and Performance) session	Written/viva voce/ skill assessment
CM2.3	Describe and demonstrate in a simulated environment the assessment of barriers to good health and health seeking behavior	Lecture, small group discussion, DOAP (Demonstration, Observation, Assistance and Performance) session	Written/viva voce/ skill assessment
PE8.4	Elicit history on the complementary feeding habits	Bedside clinics, skills lab	Skill assessment
PE8.5	Counsel and educate mothers on the best practices in complimentary feeding	DOAP (Demonstration, Observation, Assistance and Performance) session	Document in log book

7.1 Information Regarding Customs and Health Practices

7.1.1 Menstrual Health

1. Menstruation is a normal physiological process: ☐ Yes/☐ No

2. Any food restrictions followed during menstruation: ☐ Yes/☐ No

3. Any other restrictions during menstruation: (Custom/Religious)   ☐ Yes/☐ No;
   Restrictions on movement in and out of the house   ☐ Yes/☐ No

7.1.2 Marriage

1. What is the legal age for marriage in India for boys ...., for girls ....

2. At what age were you married? ....

3. In your opinion, what should be the age for marriage in boys .... years, and in girls .... years.

7.1.3 Child Bearing (Antenatal)

1. Age of the mother at the birth of first child ....

2. Number of children born:...

3. Age at last pregnancy: ....

   Details regarding the last pregnancy and its outcome:

   a. Registered in antenatal clinic: ☐ Yes/☐ No

      If yes, in which month (*period of gestation*) ....

   b. Received antenatal care: ☐ Yes/☐ No...

   c. Number of antenatal visits ....

   d. Whether food intake increased: ☐ Yes/☐ No

   e. Any food restriction: .... ☐ Yes/☐ No

      If yes, mention...

   f. Any special/additional food item given?   ☐ Yes/☐ No, If yes, mention ....

   g. Number of hours of rest in daytime: ☐ Nil/...

   h. Any complications during pregnancy: ☐ Yes/☐ No If yes,...

   i. Anemia :☐ Present/ ☐ Absent (as per record/history)

   j. Outcome of pregnancy: ☐ Abortion/☐ Stillbirth/☐ Preterm/☐ Full term

   k. Delivery: Institutional/Home, Delivered by :☐ Doctor/☐ Nurse/☐ Trained Dai/☐ Untrained Dai/☐ Relatives or neighbours/☐ Self

   l. Cord applicants :☐ Ash/☐ Cowdung/☐ Ghee/☐ Antiseptic/☐ Other ..../none applied

   m. No. of days of isolation during puerperium:...

7.1.4 Child Rearing (Postnatal)

a. Colostrum given to newborn?   ☐ Yes/☐ No and

   Why/Why not?..

b. Breastfeeding started within how many hours and why? ....
   ....

c. Any prelacteal feeds given to the child and why? ....
   ....

d. Do you give any other food than breast milk before six months of age?   ☐ Yes/☐ No and

   why/ why not..

e. Do you give water to a child before six months?   ☐ Yes/☐ No...

f. At what age complementary feeding should be started? ....

g. When did you start complementary foods for your child? ....

h. Is your child vaccinated for the vaccines due for date?   ☐ Yes/☐ No

   If no, reasons ....

i. Did your child ever suffer from diarrhea?   ☐ Yes/☐ No

If yes, what actions did you take:

(a) ORS given: ☐ Yes/☐ No

(b) Home available fluids given: ☐ Yes/☐ No

If yes, specify ....

Any other action, specify: ....

j. Did your child ever suffer from pneumonia?   ☐ Yes/☐ No

If yes, could you recognize it?   ☐ Yes/☐ No

What were the signs and symptoms? ....

What actions did you take? ....

7.1.5 Other Child Rearing Practices

a. Application of kajal. ....☐ Yes/☐ No

If yes, with common applicator   ☐ Yes/☐ No

b. Massage with oil .... ☐ Yes/☐ No

c. Exposure to sunlight .... ☐ Yes/☐ No

d. Use of ghutti...☐ Yes/☐ No

e. Food prohibited during fever: ....☐ Yes/☐ No

f. Restrictions of fluids during diarrhea :..☐ Yes/☐ No

7.1.6 Family Planning

a. In your opinion, how many children a couple should have?...

b. What should be the gap between two children?..

c. Name contraceptive methods you know. ....

d. Which permanent sterilization methods (☐ Tubectomy/☐ Vasectomy) you will prefer and why? ....

....

e. Are you using any method of contraception?   ☐ Yes/☐ No. If yes, which one............... Since when?

f. Reasons for not using any method? ....

7.1.7 Health Seeking Behaviour

a. In case of illness, preference of health facility/facilities?   ☐ Hospital/☐ Dispensary/☐ MCH Centre/☐ Private practitioner (qualified)/☐ Private practitioner (unqualified)/☐ Any other ....

....

b. Why?...

c. Which system of medicine is preferred ?   ☐ Allopathy/☐ Homeopathy/☐ Ayurvedic /☐ Any other

Specify ....

○ **Problems identified**

- ◆ [   ]
- ◆ [   ]
- ◆ [   ]
- ◆ [   ]

○ **Advise given/action taken**

- ◆ [   ]
- ◆ [   ]
- ◆ [   ]
- ◆ [   ]

Comprehensive Management Plan (Family)

Levels of prevention	Primary: Health promotion and specific protection	Secondary: Early diagnosis and adequate treatment	Tertiary: Disability limitation and rehabilitation
1. Individual			
2. Family			
3. Community			

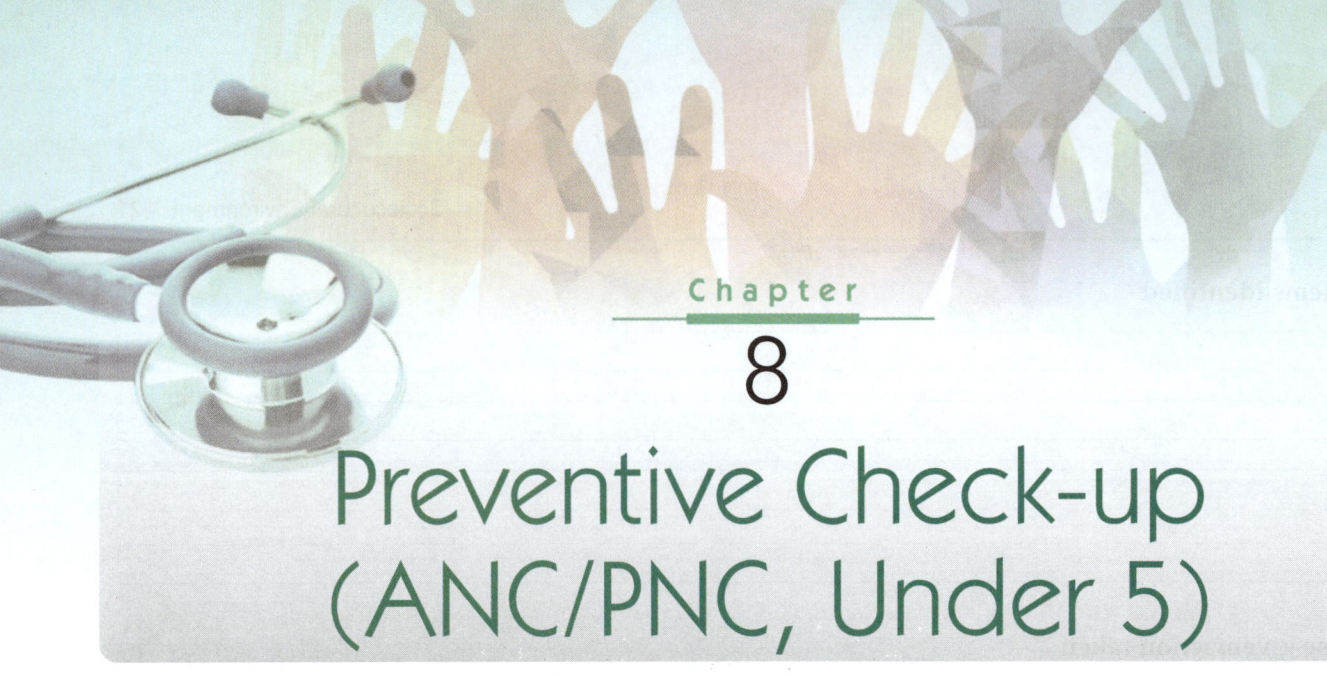

Preventive Check-up (ANC/PNC, Under 5)

8.1 Antenatal/Postnatal Check-up

Competency		Suggested teaching	Suggested assessment
CM1.9	Demonstrate the role of effective communication skills in health in a simulated environment	DOAP (Demonstration, Observation, Assistance and Performance) sessions	Skill assessment
CM1.10	Demonstrate the important aspects of the doctor–patient relationship in a simulated environment	DOAP (Demonstration, Observation, Assistance, and Performance) sessions	Skill assessment
PE18.3	Conduct antenatal examination of women independently and apply the at-risk approach in antenatal care	Bedside clinics	Skill station
PE18.6	Perform postnatal assessment of newborn and mother, provide advice on breastfeeding, weaning and on family planning	Bedside clinics, skill lab	Skill assessment
OG19.2	Counsel in a simulated environment, contraception and puerperal sterilization	DOAP (Demonstration, Observation, Assistance and Performance) session	Skill assessment

8.1.1 Identification Details

a. Name: ....

b. Age:...

c. Education: ....

d. Occupation ....

e. Parity: Gravida-primigravida/Multigravida: Parity......, Stillbirth................, Abortion........., Live............

f. Husband details:

Education: .... Occupation ....

Income ....

8.1.2 Socioeconomic Status

a. Occupation of head of household ....

b. Education of head of household ....

c. Family income: Per capita income:...(APL/BPL) ....

d. Socioeconomic status: ....

8.1.3 Clinical History

1. Chief complaints:

   a. Amenorrhea (details)..

   b. Pedal edema: ☐ Yes/☐ No

   c. Blurring of vision: ☐ Yes/☐ No

   d. Palpitation: ☐ Yes/☐ No

   e. Bleeding p/v: ☐ Yes/☐ No

   f. Discharge p/v: ☐ Yes/☐ No

2. History of present pregnancy:

   a. Conceived spontaneously: ☐ Yes/☐ No

   b. Diagnosis of pregnancy: Urine pregnancy test (UPT)   ☐ Yes/☐ No

      If yes: Self/Clinic ....

   c. ANC registration at   ☐ PHC/ ☐ Govt./ ☐ Pvt. Hospital

   d. No. of ANC visits: *(Minimum 4)*

3. Trimester history

  ○ **Trimester 1**

   a. Excessive vomiting   ☐ Yes/☐ No

   b. Bleeding p/v   ☐ Yes/☐ No

   c. Fever with rashes   ☐ Yes/☐ No

   d. Drug intake: ☐ Yes/☐ No

   e. Weight gain: *(Minimum 1 kg)*   ☐ Yes/☐ No

   f. Investigations: ☐ Hb   ☐ Blood group   ☐ RBS   ☐ VDRL

      ☐ Hep-B   ☐ HIV   ☐ Urine albumin and sugar

   g. Folate supplementation: ☐ Yes/☐ No

   h. Tetanus immunization: ☐ Yes/☐ No

  ○ **Trimester 2**

   a. Quickening: ☐ Yes/☐ No

   b. Weight gain: *Minimum 5 kg*   ☐ Yes/☐ No

   c. Blurring of vision   ☐ Yes/☐ No

   d. Epigastric pain   ☐ Yes/☐ No

   e. Pedal edema   ☐ Yes/☐ No

   f. Headache   ☐ Yes/☐ No

g. Iron folic acid supplementation: ☐ Yes/☐ No

h. Side effects (IFA supplementation)

☐ Nausea; ☐ Vomiting; ☐ Loss of appetite; ☐ Change in the colour of stools: ☐ Yes/☐ No

i. Tetanus toxoid immunization: ☐ Yes/☐ No

j. Investigations: ☐ Hb, ☐ USG

o **Trimester 3**

a. Weight gain: *(Minimum 5 kg)*

b. Warning signs

i. Pain abdomen: ☐ Yes/☐ No

ii. Decreased perception of fetal movements ☐ Yes/☐ No

iii. Leaking/Bleeding PV ☐ Yes/☐ No

4. Menstrual history:

a. Age at menarche ....

b. Regularity of the cycles: ☐ Yes/☐ No

c. Normal days of flow...

d. Excessive bleeding/clots: ☐ Yes/☐ No

e. Pain during periods: ☐ Yes/☐ No

5. Marital history:

a. Age at marriage...

b. Consanguineous/ Non-consanguineous: ☐ Yes/☐ No

c. Contraceptive usage: ☐ Yes/☐ No

6. Obstetric history:

S.No	Type of delivery	Place of delivery	Gender and weight of baby, whether cried immediately or not	Postnatal: Fever, foul smelling, lochia, bleeding PV	Feeding history Time of starting; Prelacteal feed; Duration of EBF; Complementary feed started	Present status: Immunization and nutritional status

7. Dietary history: (24 hr recall)

a. Breakfast:

b. Lunch:

c. Evening snacks:

d. Dinner:

Calories estimated: .... Calories required: .... Deficit or Excess (%) ....

Protein estimated:......................... Protein required:...................... Deficit or Excess (%)........................

8. Past history:

    a. Hypertension   □ Yes/□ No

    b. Diabetes mellitus   □ Yes/□ No

    c. Tuberculosis   □ Yes/□ No

    d. Blood transfusion   □ Yes/□ No

9. Family history:

    a. History of twins   □ Yes/□ No

    b. Preterm   □ Yes/□ No

    c. Abortion   □ Yes/□ No

10. Personal and social history:

    a. Appetite ....

    b. Sleep ....

    c. Addictions ....

    d. Family support..

11. Occupational history: ....

12. Environmental history: Housing condition..

13. Economic condition: Socioeconomic status..

14. Social welfare measures: JSY, anganwadi services ....

8.1.4 Physical Examination

1. General

    ○ Pallor/Icterus/JVP/Clubbing/Cyanosis/Lymphadenopathy/Oedema
    ○ Breast
    ○ Thyroid

2. Cardiovascular:...

3. Respiratory:...

4. Abdominal examination:

    Inspection

    ○ Shape of the abdomen
    ○ Symmetry
    ○ Fullness of the flanks
    ○ Striae gravidarum
    ○ Striae nigra
    ○ Scar

Palpation

- Abdominal girth
- Symphysio fundal height
- Fundal grip
- Lateral grip
- 1 pelvic grip
- 2 pelvic grip

Auscultation

- Fetal heart sound (FHS)

8.1.5 Management

1. Interventions:

   a. ICDS—Anganwadi centre: ☐ Awareness   ☐ Utilization

   Reasons for non-utilization ....

   b. Preparation for delivery: Money, vehicle, decision about place of delivery, awareness about JSY

   c. Plan for family planning—contraception ....

   d. Advice to continue IFA for 6 months after delivery ....

- **Problems identified**

  ◆ [   ]

  ◆ [   ]

  ◆ [   ]

  ◆ [   ]

- **Advise given/action taken:**

  ◆ [   ]

  ◆ [   ]

  ◆ [   ]

  ◆ [   ]

Comprehensive Management Plan (Family)

Levels of prevention	Primary: Health promotion and specific protection	Secondary: Early diagnosis and adequate treatment	Tertiary: Disability limitative and rehabilitation
1. Individual			
2. Family			
3. Community			

8.2 Under-five Child

Competency		Suggested teaching	Suggested assessment
CM1.9	Demonstrate the role of effective communication skills in health in a simulated environment	DOAP (Demonstration, Observation, Assistance and Performance) sessions	Skill assessment
CM1.10	Demonstrate the important aspects of the doctor-patient relationship in a simulated environment	DOAP (Demonstration, Observation, Assistance and Performance) sessions	Skill assessment
PE10.4	Identify children with under nutrition as per IMNCI criteria and plan referral	DOAP (Demonstration, Observation, Assistance and Performance) session	Document in log book

8.2.1 Identification Details

a. Name..

b. Sex ....

c. Date of Birth..

d. Age..

e. Informant: .... Reliability: ....

8.2.2 Socioeconomic Status

a. Occupation of head of household: ....

b. Education of head of household:..

c. Family income.................................. : Per capita income:...................................... (APL/BPL).................

Socioeconomic status: ....

8.2.3 Clinical History

1. Chief complaints: ....

2. History of presenting complaints: *Elaborate the chief complaints. Enquire about other complaints.*

   Ask about h/o

   - ARI
   - Diarrhea
   - Recurrent infections (respiratory and skin to be especially enquired)
   - Passing worms in stools
   - Decreased appetite
   - Chronic conditions (for example, TB)
   - Ear discharge
   - Contact with TB
   - Injuries
   - Frequency, duration, treatment sought and h/o admission in any illness reported
   - Treatment sought during any reported illness
     - Public/Private: Reason for preference
     - Duration of each episode
     - Medication given: If available
     - Cost of medication

3. Antenatal history:
   - If it is the first child: Duration between marriage and first conception
   - Birth spacing from previous delivery
   - Contraceptive use between deliveries: Reason for use/non-use
   - Registration: Govt./Pvt.
   - Antenatal visits: Total number of visits
   - Any illness during the antenatal period: Anemia, PIH, etc.
   - H/o hospital admission, referral
   - Complications during pregnancy like
     - Hyperemesis
     - Pre-eclampsia
     - Eclampsia
     - Infections
     - Antepartum hemorrhage
   - IFA intake

- Investigations done during pregnancy:
  - ◆ Hemoglobin estimation,
  - ◆ Blood grouping,
  - ◆ Ultrasound scanning.
- Visits by health worker during antenatal period

4. Natal history
   - Mode of delivery
   - Timing
   - Place of delivery
   - Birth weight
   - Complications at the time of birth
   - Cry after birth
   - Prelacteal feeds
   - Time of starting breastfeeding
   - Admission in NICU, if any and reason for admission
   - Time of discharge from the hospital
   - Postnatal visits by health worker

5. Developmental history
   a. Gross motor
   b. Fine motor
   c. Language
   d. Personal social

6. Immunization history: Vaccines given appropriate for age: ☐ Yes/ ☐ No

   Source of immunization history: Preferably immunization card

7. Nutrition history:
   - Time of starting breastfeeding after birth
   - Frequency of feeds
   - Duration of breastfeeding both exclusive and total
   - H/o administration of pre-lacteal feed
   - Time of complementary feeding and started with what items
   - Frequency of complementary feeds
   - Whether child given any commercially available preparation
   - Use of bottle feed

o 24-hour diet recall:

   a. Breakfast

   b. Lunch

   c. Evening snacks

   d. Dinner

o Calories and protein calculation:

   ♦ Required

   ♦ Actually consumed

   ♦ Deficit/excess (%)

8. Utilization of anganwadi services

   o For mother

   o For child

     ♦ Growth monitoring

     ♦ Pre-school education

     ♦ Supplementary nutrition

9. Cultural beliefs on food

   o Prelacteal feeds

   o Foods avoided in general/during illness

10. Treatment history: Undergoing any treatment for chronic condition, for the present condition, h/o treatment in the past, past hospitalisation.

11. Family history:

   o H/o chronic condition in the family especially tuberculosis

   o H/o other children of the family

   o H/o contraception usage by the couple

   o H/o smoking in the family

   o Caretaker in the absence of the mother:

     ♦ Crèche or grandmother

     ♦ Support from other family members in taking care of the child

   o Looking after the child in mother's absence

   o Accompanying to the hospital

   o Financial aid

8.2.4 General Physical Examination

Pallor/icterus/JVP/clubbing/cyanosis/lymphadenopathy/oedema

8.2.5 Anthropometry

Parameter	Observed	Expected	Deficit
Weight			
Height			
MUAC			

Reference weights for children up to five years (kg)					What should be the weight of children up to five years? (kg)				
Age (month)	Boy		Girl		Age (month)	Boy		Girl	
	If less than this, then it is low weight	Ideal weight (kg)	If less than this, then it is low weight	Ideal weight (kg)		If less than this, then child is stunted	Ideal height (cm)	If less than this, then child is stunted	Ideal height (cm)
0	2.5	3.3	2.4	3.2	0	46.1	49.9	45.4	49.1
3	5	6.4	4.5	5.8	3	63.3	67.6	61.2	65.7
6	6.4	7.9	5.7	7.3	6	63.3	67.6	61.2	65.7
9	7.1	8.9	6.5	8.2	9	67.5	72.0	65.3	70.1
12	7.7	9.6	7.0	8.9	12	71.0	75.7	68.9	74.0
15	8.3	10.3	7.6	9.6	15	74.1	79.1	72.0	77.5
18	8.8	10.9	8.1	10.2	18	76.9	82.3	74.9	80.7
21	9.2	11.5	8.6	10.9	21	79.4	85.1	77.5	83.7
24	9.7	12.2	9.0	11.5	24	81.7	87.8	80.0	86.4
27	10.1	12.7	9.5	12.1	27	83.1	89.6	81.5	88.3
30	10.5	13.3	10.0	12.7	30	85.1	91.9	83.6	90.7
33	10.9	13.8	10.4	13.4	33	86.9	94.1	85.6	92.9
36	11.3	14.3	10.8	13.9	36	88.7	96.1	87.4	95.1
39	11.6	14.8	11.2	14.4	39	90.3	98.0	89.2	97.1
42	12	15.3	11.6	15	42	91.9	99.9	90.9	99.0
45	12.4	15.8	12.0	15.5	45	93.5	101.6	92.5	100.9
48	12.7	16.3	12.3	16.1	48	94.9	103.3	94.1	102.7
51	13.1	16.8	12.7	16.6	51	96.4	105.0	95.6	104.5
54	13.4	17.3	13.0	17.2	54	97.8	106.7	97.1	106.2
57	13.7	17.8	13.4	17.7	57	99.3	108.3	98.5	107.6
60	14.1	18.3	13.7	18.2	60	100.7	110.0	99.9	109.4

Reference weight and height/length for identifying wasting

Moderate acute malnourished and severe acute malnourished table						
Length (cm)	***Boy***			***Girl***		
	Below this severe wasting (kg) (SAM)	***Between this moderate (kg) (MAM)***	***Between this normal (kg)***	***Below this severe wasting (kg) (SAM)***	***Between this moderate (kg) (MAM)***	***Between this normal (kg)***
46.0	2.0	2.0–2.1	2.2–3.1	2.0	2.0–2.1	2.2–3.2
48.0	2.3	2.3–2.4	2.5–3.6	2.3	2.3–2.4	2.5–3.6
50.0	2.6	2.6–2.7	2.8–4.2	2.6	2.6–2.7	2.8–4.0
52.0	2.9	2.9–3.1	3.2–4.5	2.9	2.9–3.1	3.2–4.6
54.0	3.3	3.3–3.5	3.6–5.1	3.3	3.3–3.5	3.6–5.2
56.0	3.8	3.8–4.0	4.1–5.8	3.7	3.7–3.9	4.0–5.8
58.0	4.3	4.3–4.5	4.6–6.4	4.1	4.1–4.4	4.5–6.5
60.0	4.7	4.7–5.0	5.1–7.1	4.5	4.5–4.8	4.9–7.1
62.0	5.1	5.1–5.5	5.6–7.7	4.9	4.9–5.2	5.3–7.7
64.0	5.5	5.5–5.9	6.0–8.3	5.3	5.3–5.6	5.7–8.3

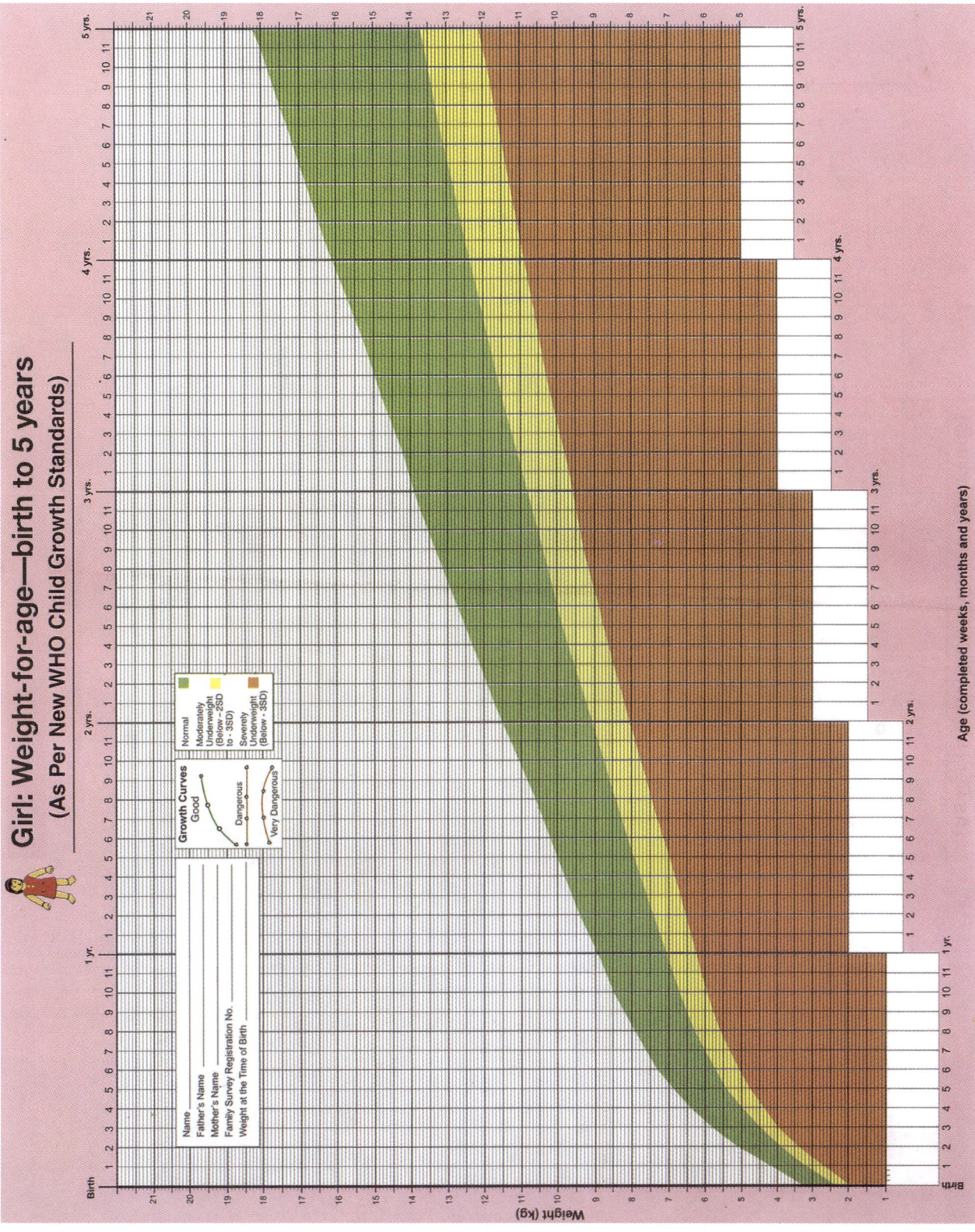

Girl: Weight-for-age—birth to 5 years
(As Per New WHO Child Growth Standards)

Growth Curves

Good

Dangerous

Very Dangerous

Normal

Moderately Underweight (Below –2SD to –3SD)

Severely Underweight (Below –3SD)

Name

Father's Name

Mother's Name

Family Survey Registration No.

Weight at the Time of Birth

Weight (kg)

Age (completed weeks, months and years)

Fig. 8.1

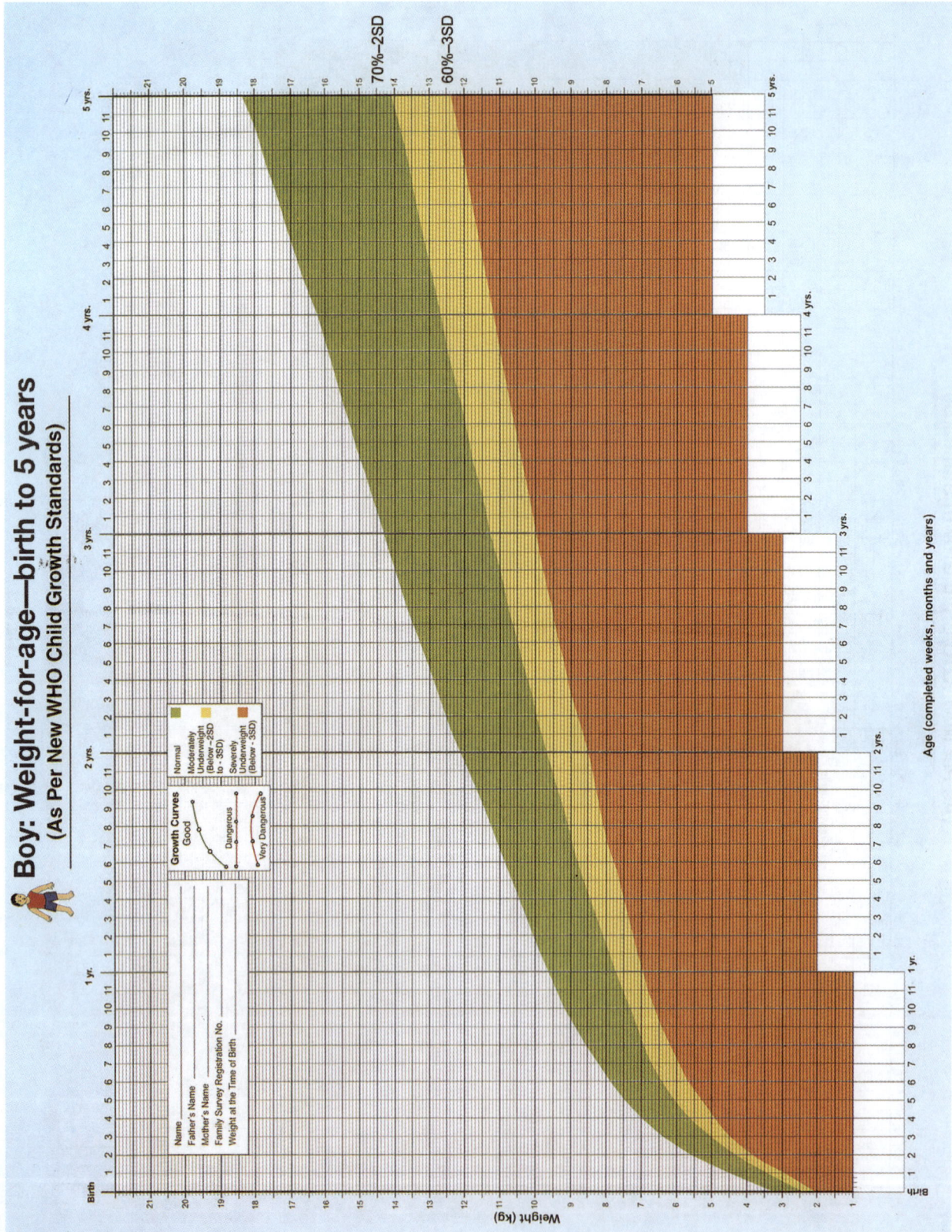

Boy: Weight-for-age—birth to 5 years
(As Per New WHO Child Growth Standards)

Fig. 8.2

8.2.6 Head to Toe Examination to Look for Evidence of Protein Energy Malnutrition

- Fontanelles, eye changes
- Skin changes: Erythema and hyperpigmentation—flaky paint dermatosis, petechiae
- Hair changes: Brittle, hypopigmented easily pluckable hair
- Nail changes: Koilonychia (iron deficiency), hypoalbuminemia

Signs of other micronutrient deficiencies:
- Vitamin A: Bitot's spots
- Vitamin D: Features of rickets like pot belly, wrist widening, rachitic rosary, bow legs, knock knees

Signs of repeated infections
- Repeated ARI: Harrison's sulcus

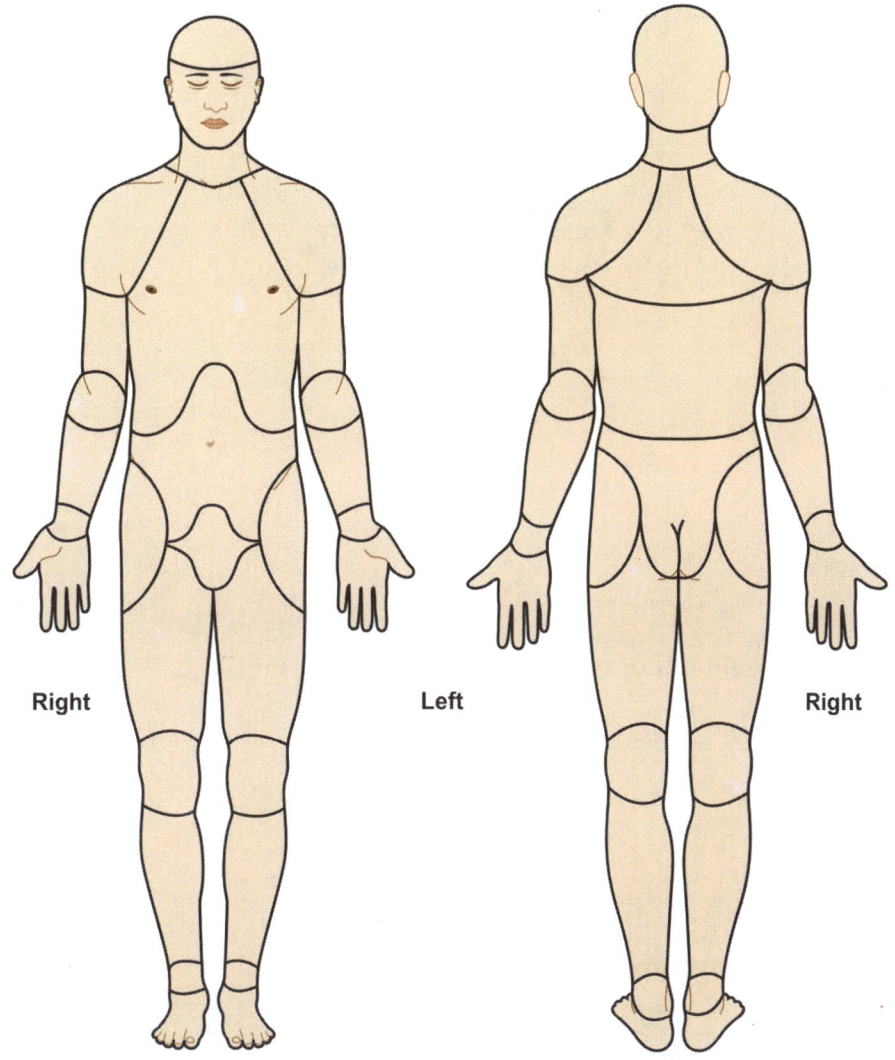

Right   **Left**   **Right**

- Repeated skin infections

8.2.7 Oral Examination

a. Dental hygiene

b. Dentition

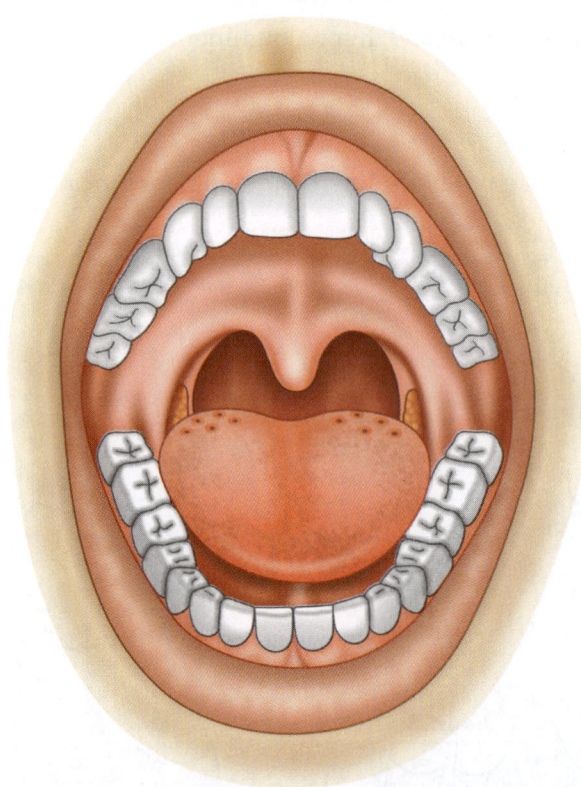

8.2.8 Systemic Examination

a. Cardiovascular system

b. Respiratory system

- ○ Wheeze: In case of current LRI or repeated LRI leading to asthma

c. Per abdomen

- ○ Hepatomegaly
- ○ Ascites

d. Central nervous system

8.2.9 Environmental History

1. Housing: Type, no. of living rooms, no. of persons, overcrowding,

2. Ventilation:
   a. Adequacy of ventilation
   b. Cross ventilation

3. Lighting

4. Drinking water: Source, storage, method of retrieval

5. Cooking fuel

   a. Major mode
   b. Presence of exhaust ventilation inside the house

6. Personal hygiene: Frequency of bathing, brushing teeth, cutting nails, practice of wearing chappal

7. Cleanliness of the house

8. Cleanliness of surrounding area: Look for possible breeding areas, garbage, etc.

9. Sanitary latrine: Present/absent

10. Drinking water supply: Any household purification method used

11. Waste disposal:

    a. Sewage, sullage and refuse

    b. Children's fecal matter

12. Pets in the house

13. Assess risk of childhood injuries

    a. Flooring: Slippery

    b. Sharp or projecting edges in the house

    c. Height of the bed

    d. Power sockets, insect repellents, kerosene, medications, etc., in reach of the child

Diagnosis

8.2.10   Management

1. Interventions:

   a. *Immediate:* Clinical management of any existing condition, deworming

   b. Dietary advice for malnourished child:

      i. Supplement deficiency in calories and proteins

         ⇒ Supplement deficiency in calories and micronutrients

         ⇒ Locally available and low cost foods

         ⇒ Food items preferred by the family and the child

      ii. Micronutrient deficiency, if exists

      iii. *Long term:* Personal hygiene, vaccination, vitamin prophylaxis, nutritional advice, weight monitoring, anganwadi service utilisation, family planning choices, importance of birthspacing.

Negative Factors

○ **Problems identified**

- [blank]
- [blank]
- [blank]
- [blank]

○ **Advise given/action taken:**

- [blank]
- [blank]
- [blank]
- [blank]

Comprehensive Management Plan (Family)

Levels of prevention	Primary: Health promotion and specific protection	Secondary: Early diagnosis and adequate treatment	Tertiary: Disability limitation and rehabilitation
1. Individual			
2. Family			
3. Community			

IMNCI (Integrated Management of Neonatal and Childhood Illnesses):

The IMNCI clinical guidelines target children less than 5 years old—the age group that bears the highest burden of deaths from common childhood diseases.

The guidelines based on evidence-based syndromic approach are used by the health worker to determine the:

- ○ Health problem(s) the child may have;
- ○ Severity of the child's condition;
- ○ Actions that can be taken to care for the child (e.g. refer the child immediately, manage with available resources, or manage at home)

The case management process is presented on a series of charts, which show the sequence of steps and how to perform them.

MANAGEMENT OF THE SICK YOUNG INFANT AGE UP TO 2 MONTHS

Name: .... Age: .... Weight: ....kg Temperature: ....°C Date ....

Ask: What are the infant's problems? ....

Initial visit? ....

Follow-up visit ....

ASSESS (Circle all signs present)   **Classify**

CHECK FOR POSSIBLE BACTERIAL INFECTION/JAUNDICE

✖ Has the infant had convulsions?

✖ Count the breaths in one minute ..... breathes per minute

✖ Repeat if elevated ... fast breathing?

✖ Look for severe chest indrawing.

✖ Look for nasal flaring.

✖ Look and listen for grunting.

✖ Look and feel for bulging fontanelle

✖ Look for pus draining from the ear.

✖ Look at the umbilicus. Is it red or draining pus?

✖ Look for skin pustules. Are there 10 or more pustules or a big boil?

✖ Measure axillary temperature (if not possible, feel for fever or low body temperature)

◊ 37.5°C or more (or feels hot)?

◊ Less than 35.5°C?

◊ Less than 36.5°C but above 35.4°C (or feels cold to touch)?

✖ See if young infant is lethargic or unconscious

✖ Look at young infant's movements. Less than normal?

✖ Look for jaundice. Are the palms and soles yellow?

Does the young infant have diarrhea?   Yes ....No...............

✖ For how long? ...... Days ☐ ☐

✖ Is there blood in the stool?

✖ Look at the young infant's general condition. Is the infant:

◊ Lethargic or unconscious?

◊ Restless and irritable?

✖ Look for sunken eyes

✖ ☐ ☐ Pinch the skin of the abdomen, Does it go back?

◊ Very slowly (longer than 2 seconds)?

◊ Slowly

Contd.

Then check for feeding problems and malnutrition

✕ If there any difficulty feeding? ☐ Yes/☐ No   Determine weight for age. Very low... low... not low...

✕ Is the infant breastfed? ☐ Yes/ ☐ No

  If yes, how many times in 24 hours? ....times

✕ Does the infant usually receive any other foods or drinks? ☐ Yes/ ☐ No

  If yes, how often?

✕ What do you use to feed the infant?

If the infant has any difficulty feeding.

Is feeding less than 8 times in 24 hours.

Is taking any other food or drinks or is low weight for age and has no indications to refer urgently to hospital:

✕ Has the infant breastfed in the previous hour?

  If infant has not fed in the previous hour, ask the mother to put her infant to the breast. Observe the breastfeed for 4 minutes.

  ◇ Is the infant able to attach? To check attachment, look for:

    ➢ Chin touching breast   ☐ Yes/☐ No

    ➢ Mouth wide open   ☐ Yes/☐ No

    ➢ Lower lip turned outward   ☐ Yes/☐ No

    ➢ More areola above than below the mouth   ☐ Yes/☐ No

           no attachment at all   not well attached   good attachment

  ◇ Is the infant suckling effectively (that is, slow deep sucks, sometimes pausing)?

           not sucking at all   not sucking effectively   sucking effectively

  ◇ Look for ulcers or white patches in the mouth (thrush).

✕ Does the mother have pain while breastfeeding? If yes, then look for:

  ◇ Flat or inverted nipples, or sore nipples

  ◇ Engorged breasts or breast abscess

Check the young infant's immunization status   Circle immunizations needed today

BCG ....   DPT 1 ....

OPV 0 ....   OPV 1 ....

HEP-B 1a ....

Return for next

immunization on:

Date: ....

Assess other problems:

MANAGEMENT OF THE SICK CHILD AGE 2 MONTHS UP TO 5 YEARS

Name: .... Age: .... Weight: ....kg Temperature: ....°C Date ....

Ask: What are the child's problems? ....

Initial visit? ....

Follow-up visit ....

ASSESS (Circle all signs present)   **Classify**

Check for General Danger Signs ✗ Not able to drink or breastfeed ✗ Vomits everything ✗ Convulsions	Lethargic or unconscious	General danger sign present? ☐ Yes/ ☐ No Remember to use danger sign when selecting classifications
Does the child have cough or difficult breathing? ☐ Yes / ☐ No ✗ For how long? .... days	✗ Count the breaths in one minute ...... breaths per minute. Fast breathing? ✗ Look for chest indrawing. ✗ Look and listen for stridor	

Does the child have diarrhea?   ☐ Yes / ☐ No
✗ For how long? ...... Days ☐ ☐
✗ Is there blood in the stool?
	✗ Look at the child's general condition. Is the child:
	  ◈ Lethargic or unconscious?
	  ◈ Restless and irritable?
	✗ Look for sunken eyes
	✗ Offer the child fluid. Is the child:
	  ◈ Not able to drink or drinking poorly?
	  ◈ Drinking eagerly, thirsty?
	✗ Pinch the skin of the abdomen. Does it go back:
	  ◈ Very slowly (longer than 2 seconds)?
	  ◈ Slowly	

Does the child have fever? (by history/feels hot/temperature 37.5°C or above) ☐ Yes / ☐ No Decide malaria risk: ☐ High ☐ Low		

Contd.

✖ Fever for how long? .... Days

✖ If more than 7 days, has fever been present every day?

✖ Has the child had measles within the last 3 months?

✖ Look and feel for stiff neck

✖ Look and feel for bulging fontanelle

✖ Look for running nose

Look for signs of measles:
✖ Generalized rash
✖ One of these: Cough, runny nose, or red eyes

Does the child have an ear problem   ☐ Yes/ ☐ No
✖ Is there ear pain?
✖ Is there ear discharge?
  If yes, for how long? .... Days

✖ Look for pus draining from the ear.
✖ Feel for tender swelling behind the ear.

Then check for malnutrition

✖ Look for visible severe wasting.
✖ Look for edema of both feet
✖ Determine weight for age
  Very low .... Not very low ....

Then check for anaemia

✖ Look for palmar pallor
  ◊ Severe palmar pallor?
  ◊ Some palmar pallor?
  ◊ No pallor?

Check the Child's Immunization, Prophylactic Vitamin A and Iron-Folic Acid Status
Circle immunizations and vitamin A or IFA supplements needed today.

BCG ....   DPT 1 ....   DPT 2 ....   DPT 3 ....   DPT (Booster)   DT ....
                                                                          ....

OPV 0 ....   OPV 1 ....   OPV 2 ....   OPV 3 ....   IFA ....
                                                         OPV ....

          HEP-B1 ....   HEP-B2 ....   HEP-B3 ....   Vitamin A

                                                 Measles ....

Return for next immunization or vitamin A or IFA supplement on:

Date: ....

Assess child's feeding if child has very low weight or anemia or is less than 2 years old
✖ Do you breastfeed your child   ☐ Yes/ ☐ No
  If yes, how many times in 24 hours? ....times.
  Do you understand during the night?   ☐ Yes/ ☐ No
✖ Does the child take any other food or fluids?   ☐ Yes/ ☐ No
  If yes, what fluids or fluids? ....
  ....
  How many times per day? ....times. What do you use to feed the child and how? ....
  How large are the servings? ....
  Does the child receive his own serving? .... Who feeds the child and how? ....
✖ During this illness, has the child's feeding changed?   ☐ Yes/ ☐ No
  If yes, how?

Assess other problems:

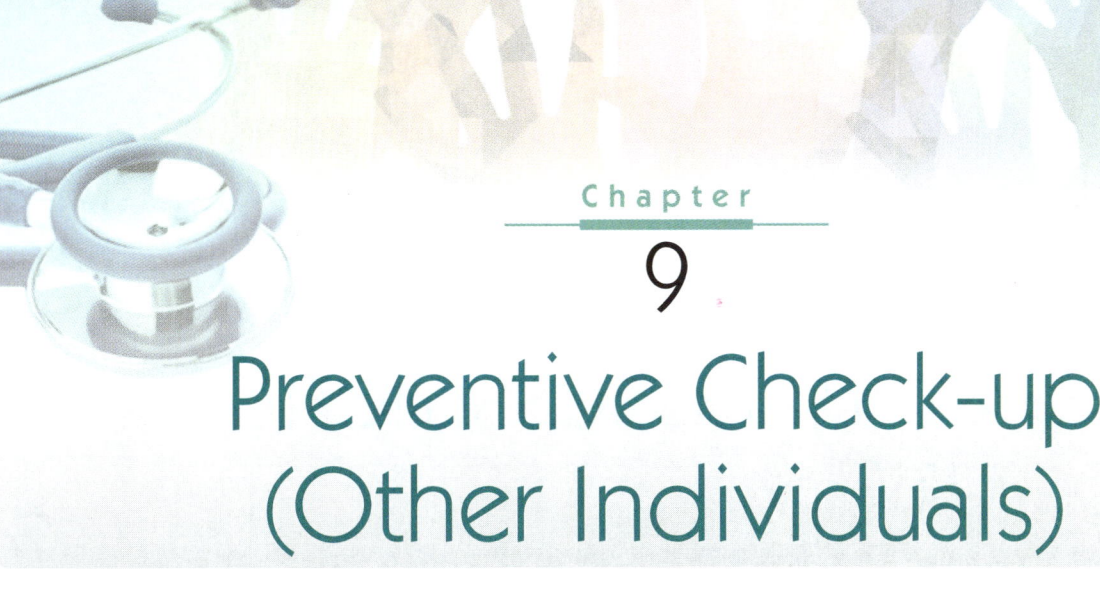

Preventive Check-up (Other Individuals)

Competency		Suggested teaching	Suggested assessment
CM1.9	Demonstrate the role of effective communication skills in health in a simulated environment	DOAP (Demonstration, Observation, Assistance and Performance) sessions	Skill assessment
CM1.10	Demonstrate the important aspects of the doctor–patient relationship in a simulated environment	DOAP (Demonstration, Observation, Assistance and Performance) sessions	Skill assessment

9.1 Enter the Relevant Information in the Format given below for each of the Individuals

Name	Age	Conditions for which individual needs to be screened	Methods of screening	Findings/ Results	Action taken

9.2 List the Medical Problems Detected

1. ....
2. ....
3. ....

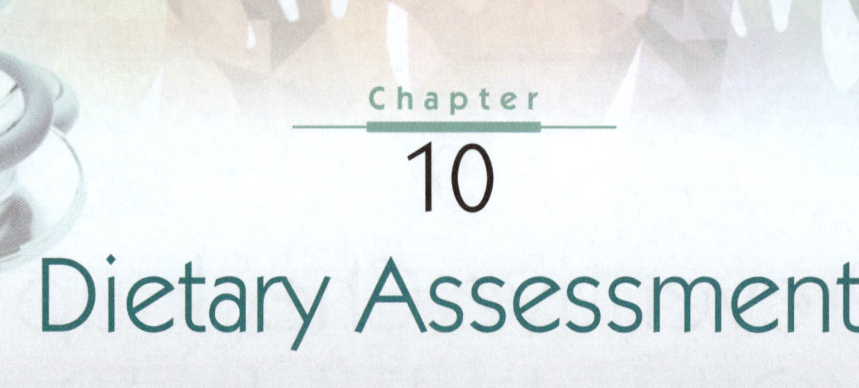

Chapter

10

Dietary Assessment

Competency		Suggested teaching	Suggested assessment
CM1.9	Demonstrate the role of effective communication skills in health in a simulated environment	DOAP (Demonstration, Observation, Assistance and Performance) sessions	Skill assessment
CM1.10	Demonstrate the important aspects of the doctor–patient relationship in a simulated environment	DOAP (Demonstration, Observation, Assistance and Performance) sessions	Skill assessment
PE9.4	Elicit, document and present an appropriate nutritional history and perform a dietary recall	Bedside clinic, skill lab	Skill assessment
PE9.5	Calculate the age-related calorie requirement in health and disease and identify gap	Bedside clinics, small group discussion	Skill assessment

10.1   Calorie Chart of Common Indian Foods

Calorie-sheet					
Item	**Quantity**	**Caloric value**	**Item**	**Quantity**	**Caloric value**
Breakfast			**Beverages**		
Egg boiled	1	80	Tea, black, no sugar	1 cup	10
Egg fried	1	110	Coffee, black, no sugar	1 cup	10
Egg omelette	1	120	Tea with milk and sugar	1 cup	45
Bread slice with butter	1	90	Coffee, milk and sugar	1 cup	45
Chapati	1	60	Milk without sugar	1 cup	60
Puri	1	75	Milk with sugar	1 cup	75
Paratha	1	150	Horlicks, milk and sugar	1 cup	120
Sabji	1 cup	150	Fresh fruit juice	1 cup	120

Contd.

Calorie-sheet (*Contd.*)					
Item	*Quantity*	*Caloric value*	*Item*	*Quantity*	*Caloric value*
Idli	1	100	Aerated soft drinks	1 bottle	90
Dosa plain	1	120	Beer	1 bottle	200
Dosa masala	1	250	Soda	1 bottle	10
Sambhar	1 cup	150	Alcohol, neat	1 peg, small	75
Lunch/Dinner			**Miscellaneous**		
Cooked rice, plain	1 cup	120	Jam	1 tsp	30
Cooked rice, fried	1 cup	150	Butter	1 tsp	50
Phulka	1	60	Ghee	1 tsp	50
Nan	1	150	Sugar	1 tsp	30
Dal	1 cup	150	Biscuit	1	30
Curd	1 cup	100	Fried nuts	1 cup	300
Curry, vegetable	1 cup	150	Puddings	1 cup	200
Curry, meat	1 cup	175	Ice-cream	1 cup	200
Salad	1 cup	100	Milk shake	1 glass	200
Papad	1	45	Wafers	1 pkt	120
Cutlet	1	75	Samosa	1	100
Pickle	1 tsp	30	Bhel puri/pani puri	1 helping	150
Soup, clear	1 cup	75	Kabab	1 plate	150
Soup, heavy	1 cup	50	Indian sweet/mithai	1 pc	150
			Fruit	1 helping	75

10.2　Method for Assessment of Average Daily Energy Intake

○ Ensure the diet assessment is for a regular and typical day.

○ Take dietary history by 24-hour recall.

1. Energy requirements of Indians:

Group	Category/ Age	Body wt. (kg)	Energy (kcal/d)	Protein (g/d)
Man	Sedentary work		2320	
	Moderate work	60	2730	60
	Heavy work		3490	

Contd.

Group	Category/ Age	Body wt. (kg)	Energy (kcal/d)	Protein (g/d)
Woman	Sedentary work		1900	55
	Moderate work		2230	
	Heavy work	55	2850	
	Pregnant woman		+350	78
	Lactation 0–6 months		+600	74
	6–12 months		+520	68
Infants	0–6 months	5.4	500	1.16 g/kg/day
	6–12 months	8.4	670	1.69 g/kg/day
Children	1–3 years	12.9	1060	16.7
	4–6 years	18.0	1350	20.1
	7–9 years	25.1	1690	29.5

Total number of family members: ....

Total number of consumption units *: ....

Key for calculating consumption units:

Adult male	Sedentary: 1.0, Moderate worker: 1.2, Heavy worker: 1.6
Adult female	Sedentary: 0.8, Moderate worker: 0.9, Heavy worker: 1.2
Adolescents (12–21 yrs)	1.0
Children	9 to 12 yrs: 0.8, 7 to 9 yrs: 0.7, 5 to 7 yrs: 0.6, 3 to 5 yrs: 0.5, 1 to 3 yrs: 0.4

2. Planning an appropriate diet for any special case in the family (*malnourished child, ANC/PNC, tuberculosis, diabetes, hypertension, elderly, etc.*)

For malnourished child, ANC/PNC, tuberculosis, etc. energy intake is calculated first using 24 hour recall. After that calculate any energy deficit or excess according to age and plan diet accordingly.

For elderly, according to FAO/WHO committee, after the age of 40 years, requirements should be reduced by 5 percent each decade until age of 60, and by 10 percent for each decade thereafter.

11

Case Presentations (Diabetes, Hypertension, etc.)

Competency		Suggested teaching	Suggested assessment
CM1.9	Demonstrate the role of effective communication skills in health in a simulated environment	DOAP (Demonstration, Observation, Assistance and Performance) sessions	Skill assessment
CM1.10	Demonstrate the important aspects of the doctor–patient relationship in a simulated environment	DOAP (Demonstration, Observation, Assistance and Performance) sessions	Skill assessment

List of Important Cases

a. Normal under-five child

b. Under-five child with PEM/vitamin A deficiency/worm infestation/ARI/anemia/diarrhea/CSOM, application of IMNCI strategy to under-five sick child, etc.

c. Normal ANC/ANC with anemia/BOH/medical problems, e.g. diabetes/pre-eclampsia /hypertension, etc.

d. Postnatal case: Normal/with complications

e. Couple with infertility/family planning issues

f. Communicable diseases, e.g. tuberculosis, leprosy, scabies, malaria, poliomyelitis, typhoid, hepatitis, measles, chickenpox, etc.

g. Non-communicable diseases, e.g. hypertension, diabetes, cataract, CAD, stroke, bronchial asthma, COPD, problems of geriatric age group, cancers, RHD, etc.

h. Nutritional disorders: Anemia, undernutrition, obesity, goitre, rickets, etc.

i. Person living with AIDS

j. Other problems: Incomplete immunization, environmental problems, sociocultural problems, drug dependence and alcoholism, broken family, mental health problems, psychosocial problems, etc.

Case 1: Diabetes Mellitus

1. Brief information about the reference person

   Name..

   Age...Gender...

   Occupation..Income...

   Education.. Socioeconomic status...

   Address..

2. Details of family members

3. Chief complaints

4. H/o presenting illness: Pertaining to DM-

   Describe onset, progression and treatment availed in chronological order:

   ○ Reasons for delay in seeking treatment ....

   ○ Failure of early diagnosis, treatment ....

   ○ Places of treatment (when, where, how it was diagnosed, which symptom made him seek consultation and what health education was provided about—diet/follow-up investigations/foot exam/foot care)

   ....

   ....

   ....

   ○ Treatment drugs details, regular or not..

   ○ Side effects of drugs   □ Yes/□ No

   ○ Reasons for different places of treatment, satisfaction with services

   ○ Number of consultations...

   ○ Frequency of follow-up/investigations

   ○ Any referrals   □ Govt/□ Pvt

   ○ H/o use of other systems of medicine for treatment: AYUSH

   Complications (if any): Type, who noticed, how did it manifest, what was he/she advised?

   ....

   ....

Microvascular

○ H/o blurring of vision/progressive loss of vision: Acuity/floaters/distortion/double vision/pain eyes (retinopathy)

○ H/o decreased urine output/frothing of urine/edema legs/face (nephropathy)

○ H/o burning sensation/numbness/tingling/sharp pains in lower limbs/foot ulcers (neuropathy)

○ Recurrent vomiting/ urge to pass feces after food intake/recurrent episode of loose stools (gastroparesis —autonomic neuropathy)

○ H/o postural hypotension (autonomic dysfunction)

Macrovascular

- H/o weakness in limbs/facial muscles (stroke)
- H/o chest pain as with sweating/palpitation/syncope/dyspnea on exertion (myocardial)
- Pain during walking—intermittent claudication pain in lower limbs (atherosclerosis)

Infections

- Recurrent dysuria (UTI)...
- H/o skin abscess/skin ulcers...
- H/o ear pain/ear discharge (malignant otitis externa) ....
- H/o tooth pain/foul odour from mouth (dental abscess) ....
- Persistent cough with expectoration/foul smelling sputum (pneumonia) ....

Diabetic Ketoacidosis Symptoms

- Nausea/vomiting
  - Thirst/polyuria
  - Abdominal pain
  - Shortness of breath

Past History

- H/o viral infections, surgeries, major trauma, blood transfusions ....
- H/o autoimmune diseases ....
- H/o drug intake: Diabetogenic drugs/steroids/thiazide diuretics ....
- History of cardiovascular disease...
- H/o hypertension/heart disease/known kidney disease/tuberculosis.................................

Personal History

- Addictions: Smoker/alcohol/tobacco/drugs ....
- Sleep/appetite...
- Bowel and bladder habits ....
- Hygiene..
- Physical activity ....

Menstrual History

Marital Status

Antenatal History

History of gestational diabetes mellitus or delivery of baby >4 kg (9 lb)/recurrent fetal loss

Family History

a. Family type ....

b. Family H/o DM/HTN/Heart disease/kidney disease/paralysis ....

c. List of morbidities/complications in family ....

d. Family members screened for HTN/DM ....

e. Emotional support ....

f. Response of family towards illness, who accompanies to hospital ....

Social History

o Interaction with society

o Response of society towards person

o Stigma: Yes/No

o Participation in festivals/marriages/social activities

Environment

a. Housing ....

b. No. of living rooms ....

c. Overcrowding: P/A ....

d. Ventilation ....

e. Lighting ....

f. Cooking place/utensils/cooking gas ....

g. Toilet facilities/refuse disposal/handwashing ....

h. Methods of waste disposal/ how frequently cleared ....

i. Drinking water supply—source/frequency/quantity/quality/frequency/storage/boiling ....

j. Animals/pets ....

k. Occupational environment (insect, if possible) ....

l. Mosquito/rats ....

m. Drains/septic tank ....

n. Outdoor space ....

Economic Conditions

a. Total family income ....

b. Expenditure on diet/medical care/recreations/education ....

c. Savings/debts ....

d. Ration card: ....

e. Aadhar card: ....

f. Cost incurred: ....

Medical Expenses

○ Consultation fee..

○ Investigation...

○ Treatment, travel, nutrition—extra care

  ♦ Any loss of wage/work

  ♦ Loss of quality of life

  ♦ Stress

Nutritional History

○ 24-hr recall dietary method ....

○ Veg/non-veg ....

○ Tabular format for breakfast, lunch, evening snacks and dinner...

○ Total daily calorie intake........................... deficient/adequate/excess ....

○ Total daily protein intake........................... deficient/adequate/excess ....

○ Fibre intake (fruits/veg) ....

○ Salt/fried food intake...

○ Refined carbohydrate intake (sugar, starchy foods) ....

○ Oil/any mixing of oil ....

○ Food beliefs/food taboos/customs ....

General and Systemic Examination

○ Conscious/oriented

○ Built/nourishment

○ Height/Weight/BMI/waist circumference/waist–hip ratio

○ Pulse rate

  ♦ Vessel wall thick (atherosclerosis)

  ♦ Radio-femoral delay

  ♦ Felt equally in all peripheral pulse (carotid/brachial/radial/fem/popliteal/dorsalis pedis/post-tibial)

○ BP

○ Pallor (in DM nephropathy): Icterus/cyanosis/clubbing/pedeal edema/general lymphadenopathy

Systemic Examination

Respiratory System

o Normal/abnormal—vesicular/bronchial

o Resonant on percussion

o Vocal resonance/fremitus

CVS

o Heart sounds/murmur

CNS

o No focal neurological deficit

o Pupil

o Consciousness

Abdomen

o P/A—soft

o Organomegaly

Special Senses

o Hearing: Tuning fork—520 Rinne test/Weber test

o Vision: Visual acuity (Snellen chart)/cataract/fundoscopy

Examination of both Knee Joints

Swelling/warmth/tender/edema

Foot Examination

o Foot sensations—monofilament

o Position sense/vibration sense/crude touch/fine touch

o Ankle jerk—present/brisk/absent

o Ulcer/wasting of muscles

Clinicosocial Diagnosis

Lab Investigations

Urine Examination

Glucose, albumin, pus cells, RBC, ketones

Blood Examination

○ Plasma glucose—fasting /postprandial

○ HbA1c

○ Urea/creatinine/Na/K

○ Lipid profile

Fundus Examination

Resting ECG

○ **Problems identified**

- ◆
- ◆
- ◆
- ◆

○ **Advise given/action taken**

- ◆
- ◆
- ◆
- ◆

Comprehensive Management Plan (Family)

Levels of prevention	Primary: Health promotion and specific protection	Secondary: Early diagnosis and adequate treatment	Tertiary: Disability limitation and rehabilitation
1. Individual			
2. Family			
3. Community			

Case 2: Hypertension (HTN)

1. Brief information about the reference person

Name...

Age...Gender...

Occupation..Income..

Education..Socioeconomic status...............................

Address..

2. Details of family members
3. Chief complaints
4. H/o presenting illness: Pertaining to HTN, Complications:
   ○ Giddiness, headache, vomiting
   ○ H/o chest pain, palpitation, tachycardia (left ventricular hypertrophy), dyspnea
   ○ H/o breathlessness immediately after lying down (orthopnea)
   ○ Visual disturbance/speech difficulties/limb weakness (cerebrovascular attack)
   ○ Decreased or increased frequency of urination, pruritus, lethargy, and weight loss, edema legs/facial puffiness, decreased urinary output (renal failure)
   ○ Visual loss/headache, H/o headache/vomiting/blurring of vision/photophobia (hypertensive retinopathy)
   ○ Panic attacks, sweating, palpitations, and abdominal cramps (pheochromocytoma)
   ○ Describe: Onset, progression and treatment availed in chronological order:
     ♦ Reasons for delay in seeking services
     ♦ Failure of early diagnosis, treatment
     ♦ Places of treatment (when, where, how it was diagnosed, which symptom made him/her seek consultation) health education/treatment—drugs regular/ not regular, side effects of drugs
     ♦ Reasons for different places of treatment, satisfaction with services, number of consultation, Frequency of follow-up/investigations, referrals
     ♦ H/o use of other systems of medicine for treatment of HTN
   ○ Complications: Type, who noticed, how did it manifest, what was he/she advised

Past History

History of DM/CAD/COPD/TB/seizure disorder/dyslipidemia, CVA, thyroid disease, kidney diseases, past surgeries, illnesses, blood transfusion/trauma

Personal History

○ Addictions: Alcohol/tobacco/drugs...

○ Sleep/appetite; bowel and bladder habits; hygiene; physical activity ....

Menstrual History

○ Menarche ....

○ Menstrual cycles ....

Marital Status

Antenatal History

o Edema legs/hypertension during pregnancy ....

Family History

Family Type

o Family h/o DM/HTN/heart disease/kidney disease/paralysis ....

o Family history of premature cardiovascular disease (men <55 years; women <65 years)..........................

o List of morbidities/complications in family ....

o Family members screened for HTN/DM ....

o Family relationships (h/o psychosocial stressors) ....

o Response of family towards illness, who accompanies to hospital ....

Social History

o Interaction with society...

o Response of society towards person...

o Stigma ....

o Participation in festivals/marriages/social activities, involvement in social groups.....................

Environment

Housing

o No. of living rooms...

o Overcrowding: P/A

o Ventilation, lighting...

o Cooking place/utensils/cooking gas ....

o Toilet facilities/refuse disposal/handwashing ....

o Methods of waste disposal/ how frequently cleared ....

o Drinking water supply: Source/frequency/quantity/quality/frequency/storage/boiling.......................

o Animals/pets, occupational environment (insect, if possible) mosquito/rats; Drains.................

Economic Conditions

1. Total family income..

2. Expenditure on diet/medical care/recreations/education..

3. Aadhar card ....

4. Cost incurred ....

Medical Expenses

- Consultation fee...
- Investigation...
- Treatment, travel, nutrition—extra care
  - Loss of wage/work
  - Loss of quality of life
  - Stress

Welfare Schemes

- Old age pension ....
- Any other details that family is availing...

Nutritional History

- 24-hr recall dietary method ....
- Veg/non-veg ....
- Tabular format for breakfast, lunch, eve snacks and dinner
- Total daily calorie intake.......deficient/adequate/excess...
- Total daily protein intake....... deficient/adequate/excess...
- Fibre intake (fruits/veg) ....
- Salt/fried food intake...
- Refined carbohydrate intake (sugar, starchy foods)...
- Oil/any mixing of oil ....
- Food beliefs/food taboos customs ....

General Examination and Systemic Examination

- Conscious/oriented...
- Built/nourishment ....
- Height/Weight/BMI/waist circumference/WHR ....
- Pulse
  - Rate/rhythm/volume/radio-femoral delay/equally felt in all peripheral vessels/vessel wall thickening
- BP: Position—sitting/lying down
  - Both limbs
  - No of readings
- Pallor/icterus/cyanosis/clubbing/edema/general lymphadenopathy

Systemic Examination

Respiratory System:

- Normal/abnormal—vesicular/bronchial...
- Percussion..
- Vocal fremitus/vocal resonance...

Cardiovascular System

- Heart sounds ....
- Murmur ....
- Apical impulse: Outwards/downwards—hyperdynamic..

CNS

- **Focal neurological deficit**
  - Power/tone
  - Deep reflexes: Biceps/triceps/supinator/knee/ankle
  - Superficial: Plantar
  - Cranial nerve examination
- **Gait**
  - No cerebellar signs: Ataxia, nystagmus, vertigo, incoordination of movements
  - Pupil: Size, symmetry, reaction to light

Special Senses

- Hearing ....
- Vision: Fundoscopy ....

Clinicosocial Diagnosis

Lab Investigations

Initial Routine

- Complete Blood Count: Total and differential
  - ESR
  - Platelet
  - Electrolytes: Na/K/Ca
- RFT: Urea/creatinine (kidney damage), uric acid, LFT, RBS

- X-ray: LVH, coarctation of aorta
- ECG: LVH features, prev MI
- Lipid profile
- Urine routine: Albumin, sugar

Follow-up

- BP monitoring ....
- Lipid profile ....
- Diabetic status..

- **Problems identified**

  -
  -
  -
  -

- **Advise given/action taken**

  -
  -
  -
  -

Comprehensive Management Plan

Levels of prevention	Primary: Health promotion and specific protection	Secondary: Early diagnosis and adequate treatment	Tertiary: Disability limitation and rehabilitation
1. Individual			
2. Family			
3. Community			

BIBLIOGRAPHY

1. Anganwadi workers manual, ICDS programme, Ministry of Women and Child Development, India
2. Calorific values of India food. Accessible from: http://indianfoodrecipeswithpictures.blogspot.com/2014/05/indian-food-calorie-counter-indianfood.html
3. Government of India, Ministry of Health and Family Welfare. IMNCI training module for physicians. Government of India, 2003.
4. ICDS growth monitoring guidelines, Ministry of Women and Child Development. Government of India. Accessible from: https://www.nipccd.nic.in/file/elearn/manual/egm.pdf
5. Joint FA. Human energy requirements. Report of a Joint FAO/WHO/UNU Expert Consultation, Rome, 17–24 October 2001.
6. Pandey VK, Aggarwal P, Kakkar R. Modified BG Prasad Socio-economic Classification, Update – 2019. Indian J Comm Health. 2019; 31, 1: 123–125.
7. POSHAN Abhiyaan Guidelines 2018, Ministry of Women and Child Development. Government of India.
8. Sheikh Mohd Saleem. Modified Kuppuswamy socioeconomic scale updated for the year 2019. Indian J Forensic Community Med 2019;6(1):1–3.

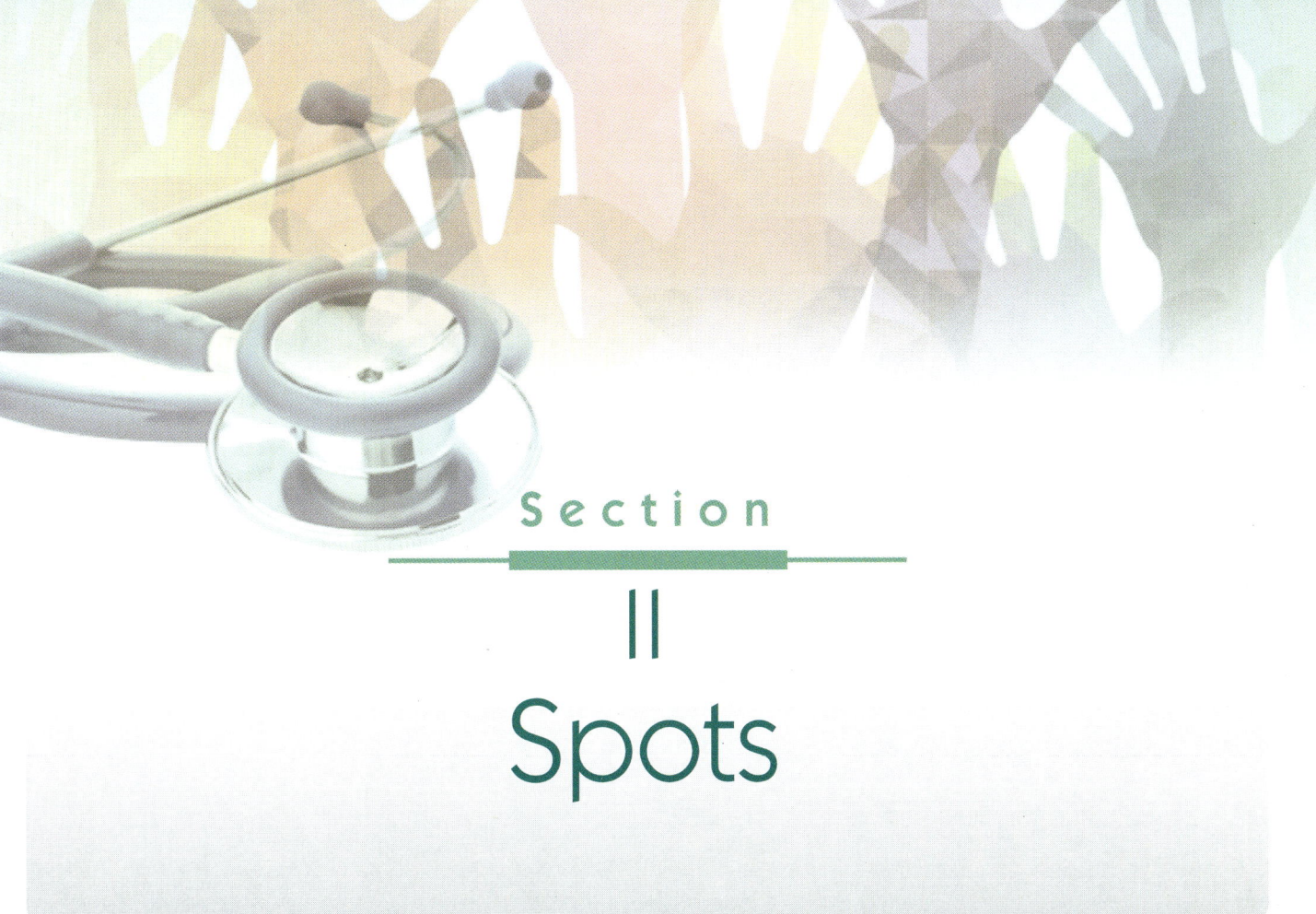

Section

II

Spots

- ◈ Cold Chain Equipment
- ◈ Vaccines
- ◈ Biomedical Waste Management
- ◈ Contraceptives
- ◈ Medicines
- ◈ Nutrition
- ◈ Entomology
- ◈ Miscellaneous

12
Cold Chain Equipment

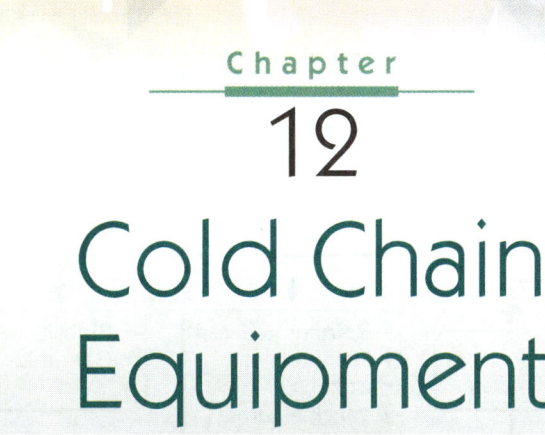

Competency		Suggested teaching	Suggested assessment
PE19.3	Vaccine description with regard to classification of vaccines, strain used, dose, route, schedule, risks, benefits and side effects, indications and contraindications	Lecture, small group discussion	Written/viva voce
PE19.4	Define cold chain and discuss the methods of safe storage and handling of vaccines	Lecture, small group discussion	Written/viva voce
PE19.4	Define cold chain and discuss the methods of safe storage and handling of vaccines	Lecture, small group discussion	Written/viva voce

Cold Chain System (Channel and Equipment)

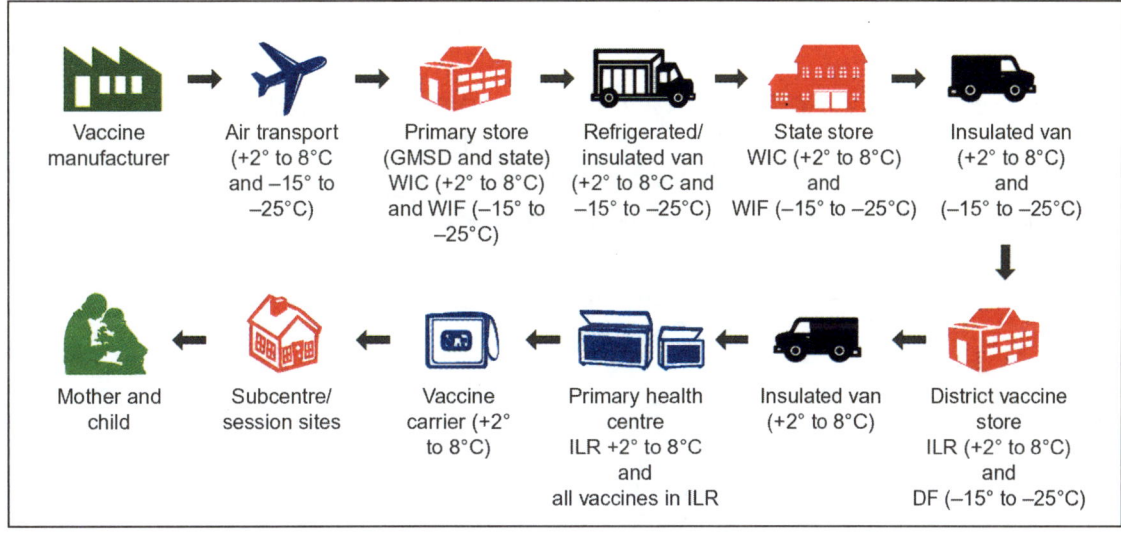

Fig. 12.1: Cold chain system

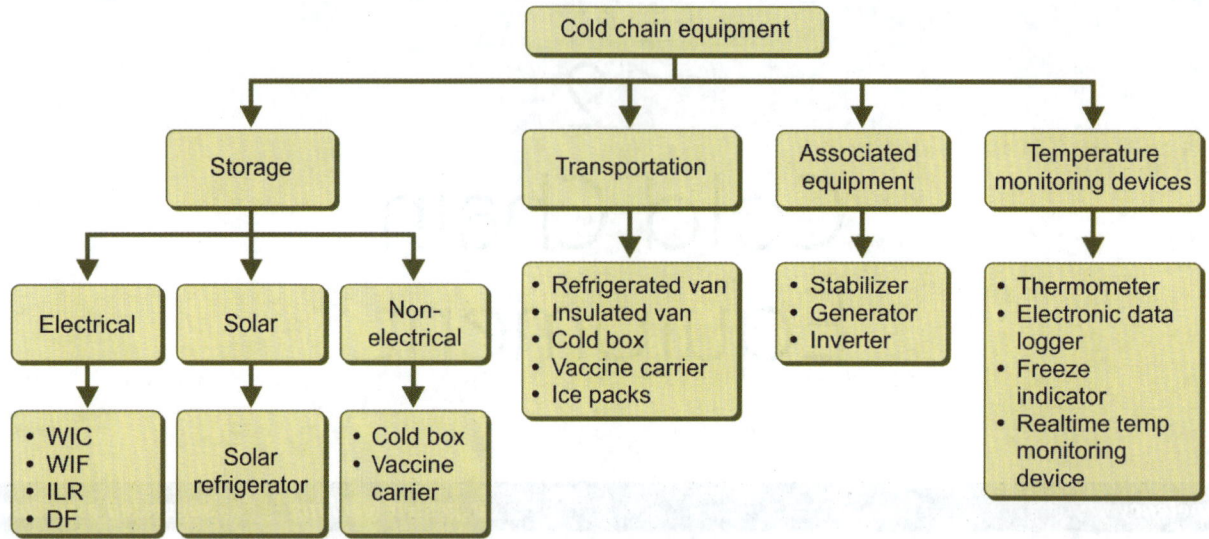

WIC—walk-in cooler; WIF—walk-in freezer; ILR—ice-lined refrigerator; DF—deep freezer

Fig. 12.2: Overview of cold chain equipment

Cold Chain Equipment (Technical Specifications)

Table 12.1: Technical specifications of cold chain equipment			
Equipment	**Temperature**	**Storage capacity**	**Holdover time**
Electrical			
Deep freezer (large)	–15° to –25°C	Ice packs or OPV stock for 3 months (275 to 300 litres)	At 43°C for 2 hrs 30 mins (minimum)
ILR (large)	+2°C to +8°C	BCG, OPV, IPV, RVV, DPT, TT, Measles/MR, Hep B, Penta, IPV, vaccine stock for 3 months (135 to 160 litres)	At 43°C for 20 hrs (minimum)
Deep freezer (small)	–15°C to –25°C	Ice packs (105 to 125 litres)	At 43°C for 2 hrs 30 mins (minimum)
ILR (small)	+2°C to +8°C	BCG, OPV, IPV, RVV, DPT, TT, Measles/MR, Hep B vaccine stocks for one month (90–105 litres)	At 43°C for 20 hrs (minimum)
Non-electrical			
Cold box (large)	+2°C to +8°C	All vaccines stored for transport or in case of power failure (20 to 25 litres)	At 43°C for 96 hrs (minimum)
Cold box (small)	+2°C to +8°C	All vaccines stored for transport or in case of power failure (5 to 8 litres)	At 43°C for 48 hrs (minimum)
Vaccine carrier (1.7 litres)	+2°C to +8°C	All vaccines carried for 12 hours (4 conditioned ice packs and 16–20 vials)	At 43°C for 36 hrs (minimum)

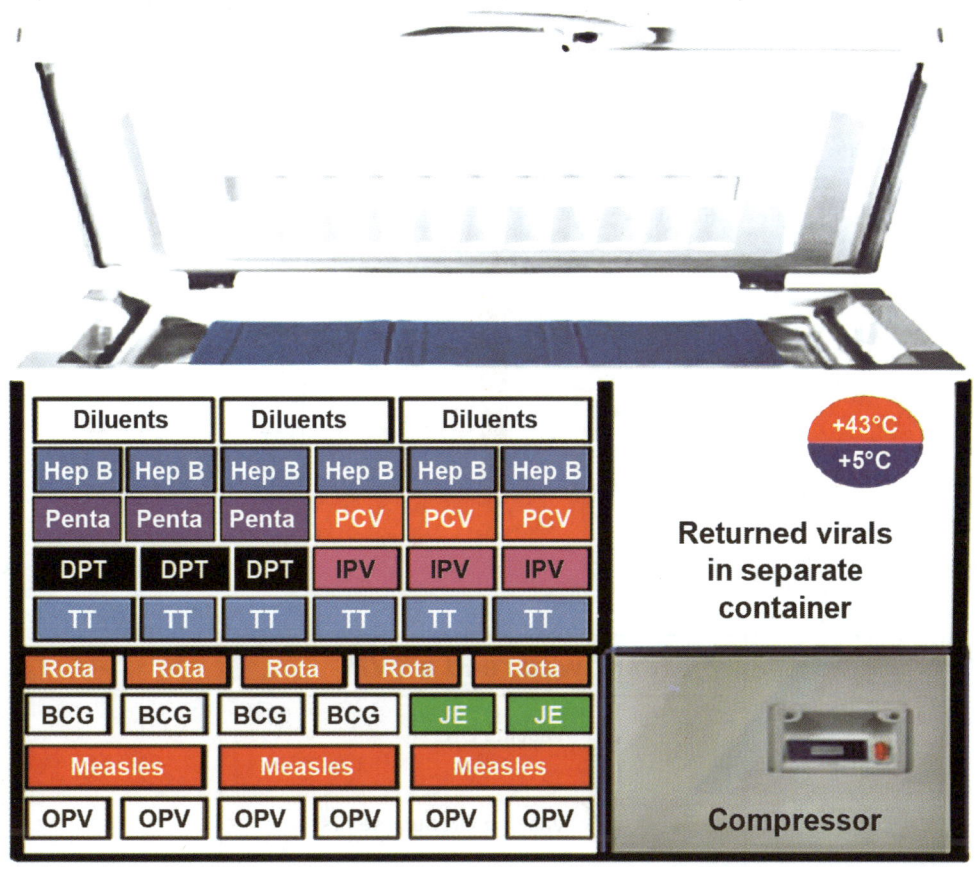

Fig. 12.3: Vaccine storage in ice lined refrigerators

Table 12.2: Sensitivity of vaccine to heat, light and freezing		
Vaccine	*Exposure to heat/light*	*Exposure to cold*
Heat and light sensitive vaccines		
OPV	Sensitive to heat	Resistant
Measles/MR	Sensitive to heat and light	Resistant
BCG, RVV and JE	Relatively heat stable, but sensitive to light	Resistant
Freeze sensitive vaccines		
Hep B/Penta/PCV	Relatively heat stable	Freezes at −0.5°C (should not be frozen)
IPV, DPT and TT	Relatively heat stable	Freezes at −3°C (should not be frozen)

Contd.

Table 12.2: Sensitivity of vaccine to heat, light and freezing *(Contd.)*

Vaccine	Exposure to heat/light	Exposure to cold
At the PHC level, all vaccines are kept in the ILR for a period of one month at temperature of +2°C to +8°C		
Vaccines sensitive to heat		Vaccines sensitive to freezing

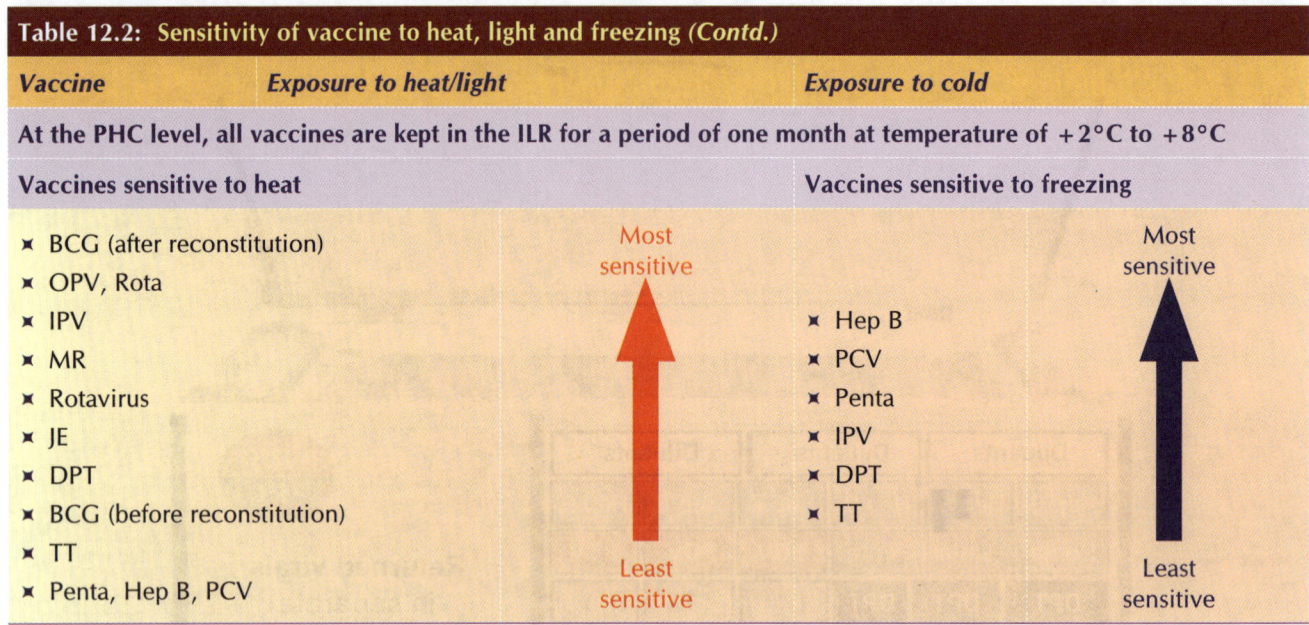

Vaccines sensitive to heat:
- BCG (after reconstitution)
- OPV, Rota
- IPV
- MR
- Rotavirus
- JE
- DPT
- BCG (before reconstitution)
- TT
- Penta, Hep B, PCV

Most sensitive → Least sensitive

Vaccines sensitive to freezing:
- Hep B
- PCV
- Penta
- IPV
- DPT
- TT

Most sensitive → Least sensitive

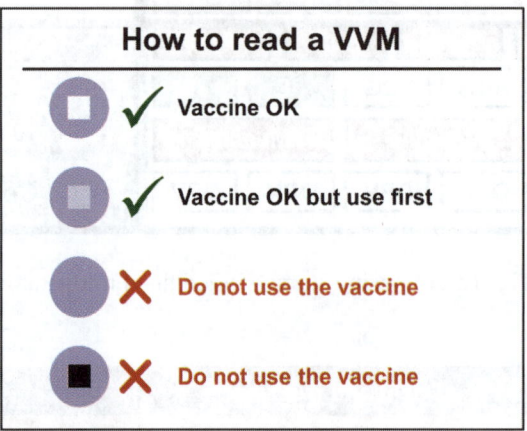

How to read a VVM

- Vaccine OK
- Vaccine OK but use first
- Do not use the vaccine
- Do not use the vaccine

Fig. 12.4: Vaccine vial monitor (instructions)

13

Vaccines

Competency		Suggested teaching	Suggested assessment
PE19.1	Explain the components of the Universal Immunization Program and the Sub-National Immunization Programs	Lecture, small group discussion	Written/viva voce
PE19.2	Explain the epidemiology of vaccine preventable diseases	Lecture, small group discussion	Written/viva voce
PE19.3	Vaccine description with regard to classification of vaccines, strain used, dose, route, schedule, risks, benefits and side effects, indications and contraindications	Lecture, small group discussion	Written/viva voce
PE19.12	Observe the administration the UIP vaccines	DOAP (Demonstration, Observation, Assistance and Performance) session	Document in log book

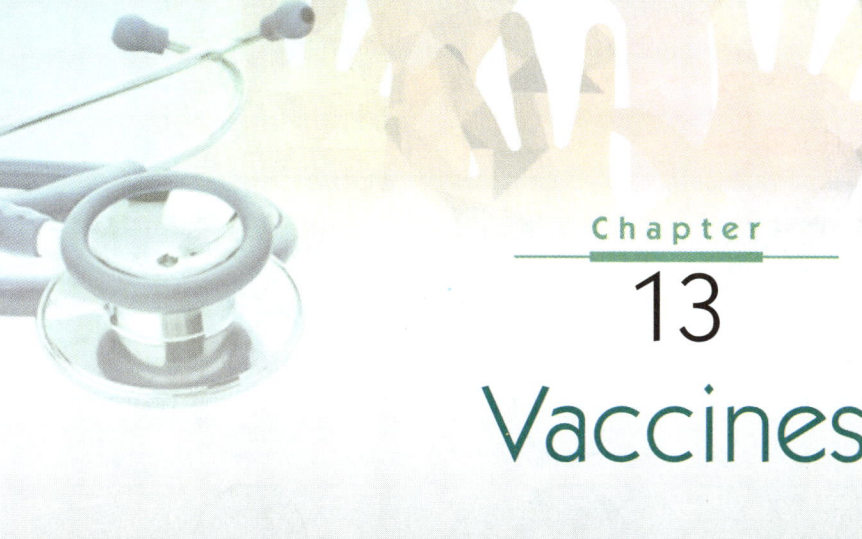

Oral administration
Oral polio vaccine — Rotavirus vaccine* — Vitamin A

Upper arm-right
IPV (intradermal) — Measles/MR* (subcutaneous)

Upper arm-left
BCG (intradermal) — JE* (subcutaneous)

Anterolateral side of mid-thigh—right (intramuscular)
PCV*

Anterolateral side of mid-thigh—left (intramuscular)
HepB birth dose — Penta — DPT booster

*Wherever applicable

Fig. 13.1: Sites of immunization under National Immunization Program

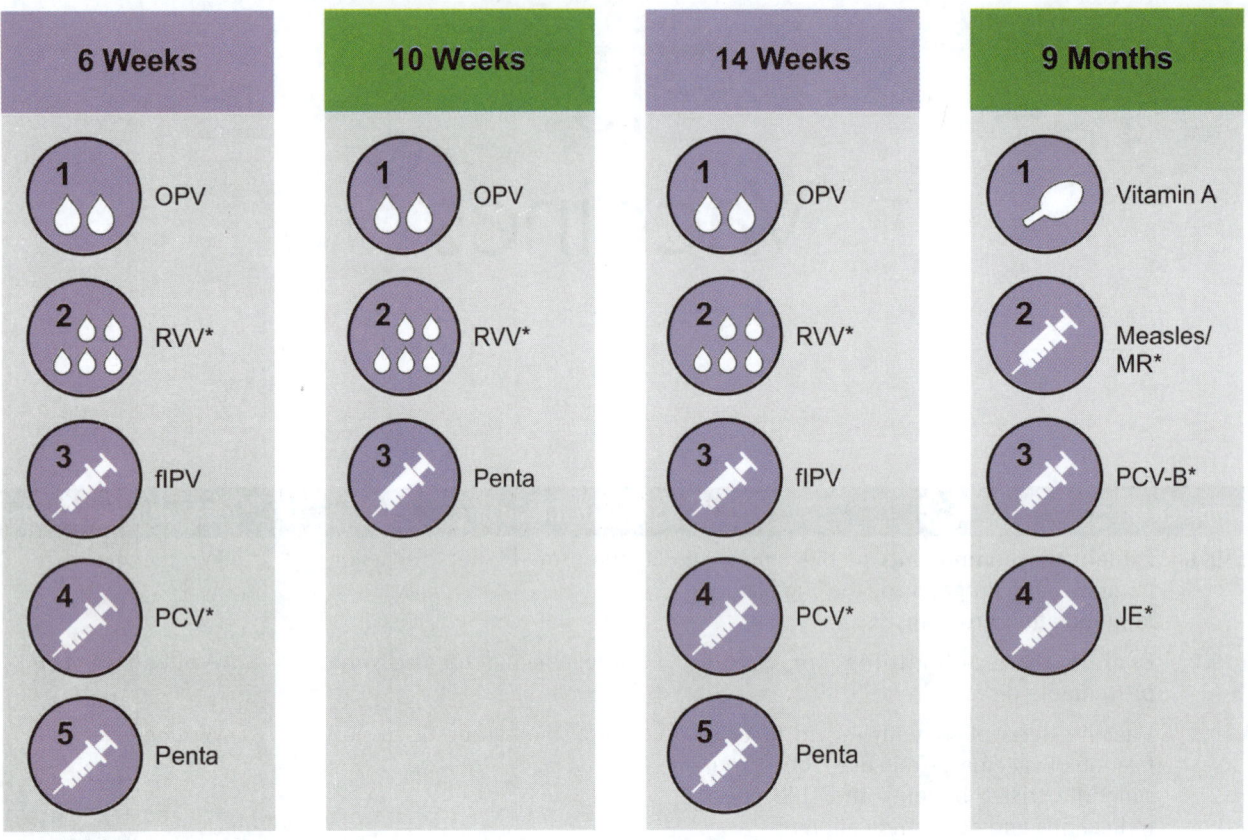

*Wherever applicable

Fig. 13.2: Schedule of vaccination under National Immunization Program (infant)

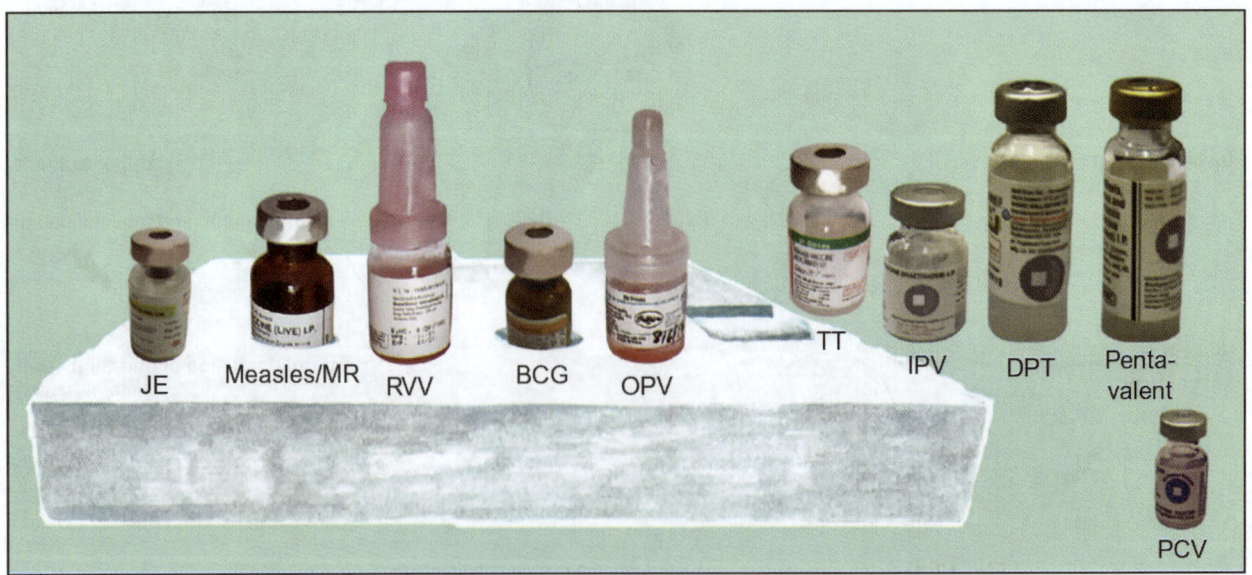

Fig. 13.3: Ice pack with positioning of vials during immunization session

Table 13.1: National Immunization Program (India)

Vaccine	Dose	Recommended age	Volume	Route and site of administration
Infants and Children				
BCG	Single	At birth	0.05 ml[1]	Intradermal (Left upper arm)
Hepatitis B	Birth dose	At birth	0.5 ml	Intramuscular (anterolateral side of left mid-thigh)
OPV	Zero dose	At birth	2 drops	Oral (mouth)
	First	6 weeks	2 drops	Oral (mouth)
	Second	10 weeks	2 drops	Oral (mouth)
	Third	14 weeks	2 drops	Oral (mouth)
	Booster	16–24 months	2 drops	Oral (mouth)
Pentavalent	First	6 weeks	0.5 ml	Intramuscular (anterolateral side of left and mid-thigh)
	Second	10 weeks	0.5 ml	Intramuscular (anterolateral side of left and mid-thigh)
	Third	14 weeks	0.5 ml	Intramuscular (anterolateral side of left and mid-thigh)
Rotavirus*	First	6 weeks	5 drops	Oral (mouth)
	Second	10 weeks	5 drops	Oral (mouth)
	Third	14 weeks	5 drops	Oral (mouth)
PCV*	First	6 weeks	0.5 ml	Intramuscular (anterolateral side of right midthigh)
	Second	14 weeks	0.5 ml	Intramuscular (anterolateral side of right midthigh)
	Booster	9 months	0.5 ml	Intramuscular (anterolateral side of right midthigh)
IPV	First	6 weeks	0.1 ml	Intradermal (right upper arm)
	Second	14 weeks	0.1 ml	Intradermal (right upper arm)
Measles/ MR*	First	9–12 months	0.5 ml	Subcutaneous (right upper arm)
	Booster	16–24 months	0.5 ml	Subcutaneous (right upper arm)
JE*[2]	First	9–12 months	0.5 ml	Subcutaneous (left upper arm)
	Second	16–24 months	0.5 ml	Subcutaneous (left upper arm)
DPT	First booster	16–24 months	0.5 ml	Intramuscular (anterolateral side of left midthigh)
	Second booster	5–6 years	0.5 ml	Intramuscular (upper arm)
TT	First	10 years	0.5 ml	Intramuscular (upper arm)
	Second	16 years	0.5 ml	Intramuscular (upper arm)
Pregnant Women				
TT	First	Earliest possible	0.5 ml	Intramuscular (upper arm)
	Second	4 weeks after 1st dose	0.5 ml	Intramuscular (upper arm)
	Booster	If received, 2 TT doses in a pregnancy within the last 3 years	0.5 ml	Intramuscular (upper arm)

1. If BCG is administered after one month of age, then dose will be 0.1 ml
2. JE vaccine is given only in endemic districts.   *Wherever applicable

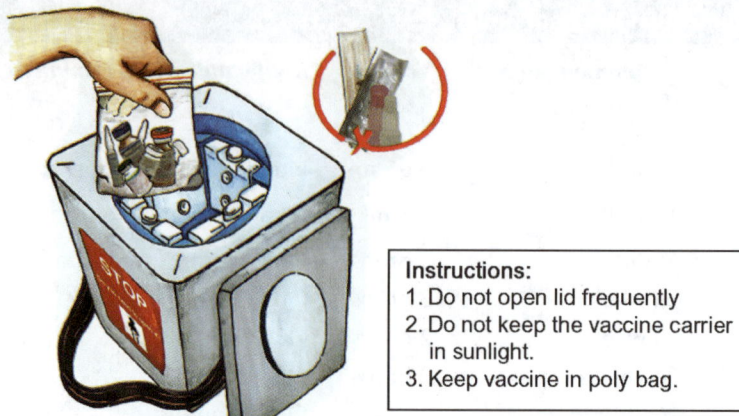

Instructions:
1. Do not open lid frequently
2. Do not keep the vaccine carrier in sunlight.
3. Keep vaccine in poly bag.

Fig. 13.4: Vaccine carrier with ice packs (precautions need to be taken while using vaccine carrier)

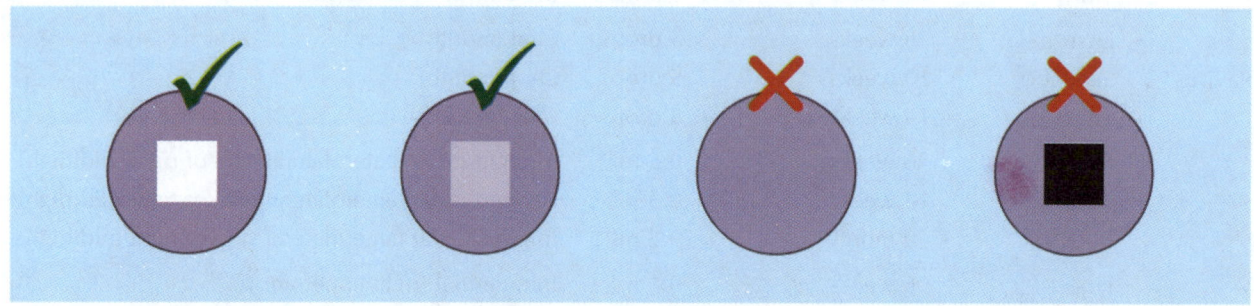

Fig. 13.5: Vaccine vial monitor

Stages of vaccine vial monitor: Stage 1 = Inner square is white; Stage 2 = Inner square is lighter than outer circle; Stage 3 = Inner square is of same color as outer circle; Stage 4 = Inner square is darker than outer circle

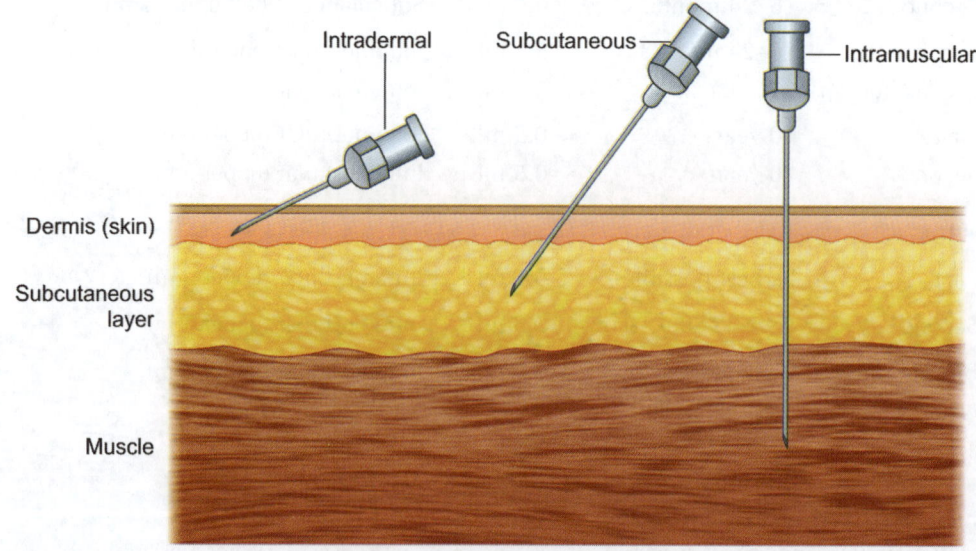

Fig. 13.6: Injection techniques

Vaccines

a. BCG and its Diluents

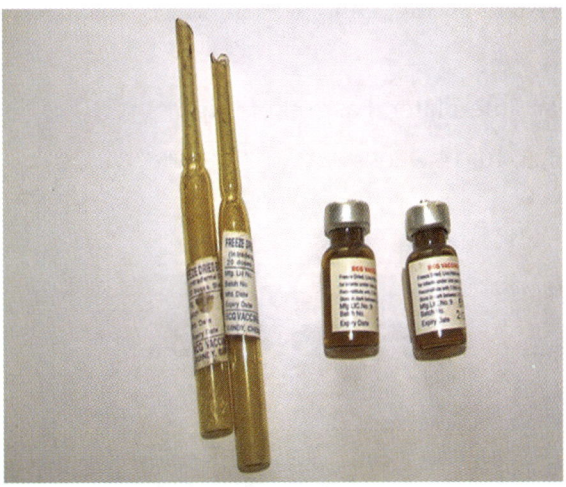

- **Composition, strain of vaccine:** Bacillus Calmette-Guérin, Danish 1331 (strain)
- **Adverse effects:** Suppurative lymphadenitis, local site reactions, osteomyelitis, disseminated BCG.
- **Contraindications:** Pregnancy, generalised eczema, infective dermatosis, immunocompromised states
- **Normal BCG reaction:** Wheal (5 mm, immediate)>> Papule (4–8 mm, 2–3 weeks)>> Ulcer (5 weeks) >> Scar (4–8 mm, 6–12 weeks)
- **Type:** Live attenuated vaccine
- **Diluent:** Normal saline
- **Route and site:** Intradermal, left arm
- **Dosage and schedule:** At birth 0.05 ml up to 1 month: 1 year (0.1 ml)

b. Pentavalent Vaccine

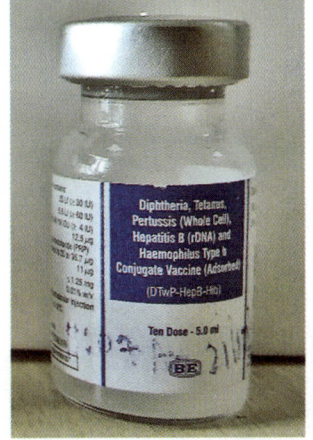

○ **Composition, strain of vaccine:** Diphtheria, pertussis, tetanus, hepatitis B, haemophilus influenzae B

○ **Adverse effects:** Local reaction, fever (pertussis component), persistent inconsolable screaming, etc.

○ **Contraindications:** Serious illness (hospital admission), neurological disorders, convulsion, severe reaction to previous dose (shock, persistent crying, etc).

○ **Type:** Killed vaccine

○ **Route and site:** Intramuscular, anterolateral aspect of thigh

○ **Dosage and schedule:** 0.5 ml, 6, 10, 14 weeks

c. DPT/DTaP/dTP

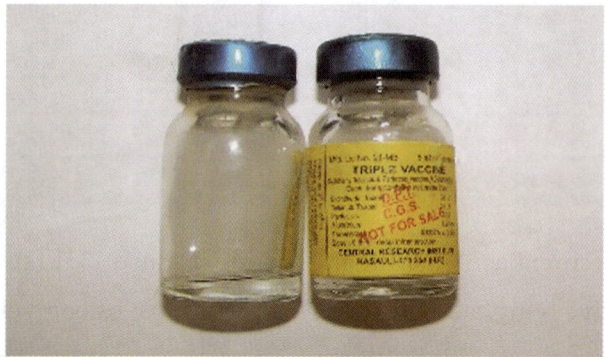

○ **Composition, strain of vaccine:** Diphtheria and tetanus (toxoid), pertussis (killed acellular bacilli)

○ **Adverse effects:** Local reaction, fever (pertussis component), persistent inconsolable screaming, hypotonic-hyporesponsive episode (HHE), etc

○ **Contraindications:** Serious illness (hospital admission), neurological disorders, convulsion, severe reaction to previous dose (shock, persistent crying, etc).

○ **Type:** Killed vaccine

○ **Route and site:** Intramuscular, anterolateral aspect of thigh

○ **Dosage and schedule:** 0.5 ml, 16–24 months, 5 years (booster)

d. Hepatitis B

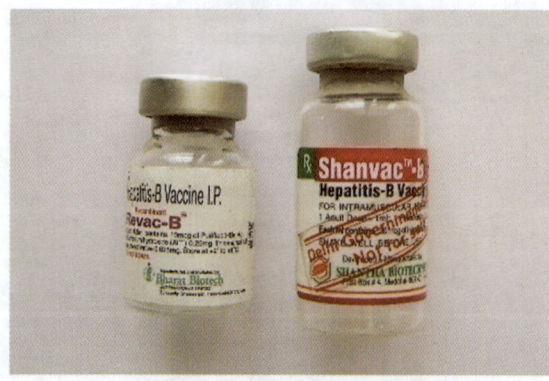

○ **Composition, strain of vaccine:** Killed recombinant type (hepatitis B virus)

○ **Adverse effects:** Local reaction

○ **Contraindications:** History of allergic reaction.

○ **Type:** Killed vaccine

○ **Route and site:** Intramuscular, anterolateral aspect of thigh

○ **Dosage and schedule:** 0.5 ml, at birth

e. Oral Polio Vaccine (OPV)

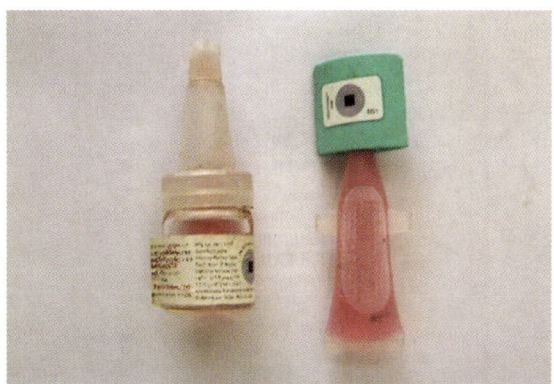

○ **Type:** Live attenuated vaccine

○ **Composition, strain of vaccine:** OPV 1,3 (bivalent)

○ **Adverse effects:** Mild diarrhea, vaccine associated paralytic polio (rare)

○ **Contraindications:** Immunocompromised state

○ **Route:** Oral

○ **Dosage and schedule:** 2 drops: At birth, 6, 10, 14 weeks

f. Injectable Polio Vaccine (IPV)

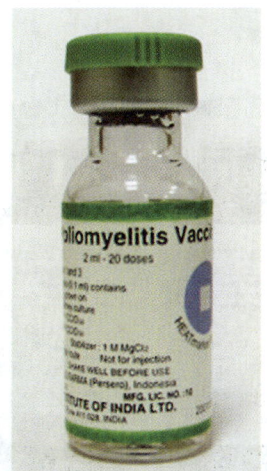

- **Type:** Killed vaccine
- **Composition, strain of vaccine:** Inactivated Polio virus (type I, II, III)
- **Adverse effects:** Local reaction
- **Contraindications:** Not suitable during epidemics
- **Route and site:** Intramuscular, anterolateral aspect of thigh
- **Dosage and schedule:** 0.5 ml, 6, 14 weeks (fractional IPV)

g. *Haemophilus Influenzae* (Hib)

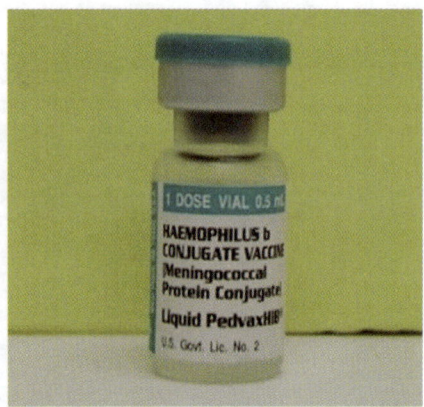

- **Type:** Killed vaccine
- **Adverse effects:** Local reaction. Fever.
- **Contraindications:** History of allergic reaction. Children less than weeks age, severe illness.
- **Route and site:** Intramuscular, anterolateral aspect of thigh
- **Dosage and schedule:** 0.5 ml, 6, 10, 14 weeks (pentavalent vaccine)

h. Measles and Diluents

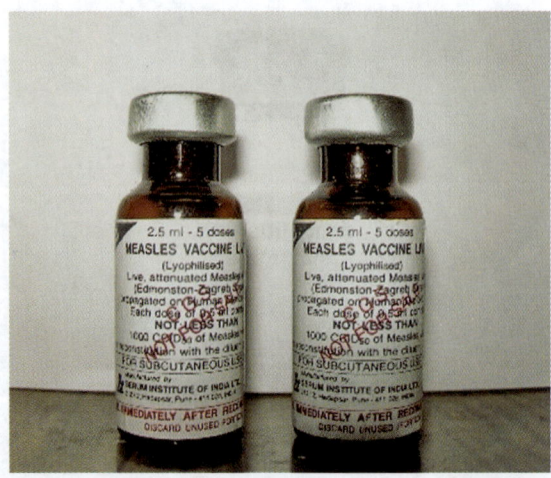

- **Type:** Live attenuated
- **Composition, strain of vaccine:** Measles: Edmonston-Zagreb strain.
- **Adverse effects:** Local reaction, toxic shock syndrome (TSS)
- **Contraindications:** High fever, serious illness, pregnant women, history of allergic reaction, immunocompromised.
- **Diluents:** Distilled water
- **Route and site:** Subcutaneous, right upper arm
- **Dosage and schedule:** 0.5 ml, 9 months (1st dose), 16–24 months (2nd dose)

i. MMR and its Diluents

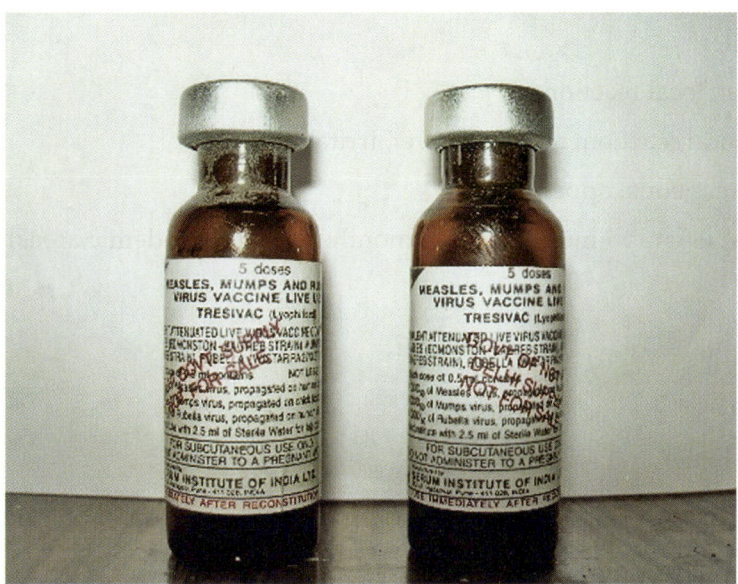

- **Type:** Live attenuated
- **Composition, strain of vaccine:** Measles (EZ strain), mumps (Jeryl-lynn) and rubella (RA 27/3)
- **Adverse effects:** TSS, arthralgia, thrombocytopenia, convulsion, encephalopathy.
- **Contraindications:** Pregnancy
- **Diluent:** Distilled water
- **Route and site:** Subcutaneous, right upper arm
- **Dosage and schedule:** 0.5 ml , 16–24 months (booster)

j. Japanese Encephalitis

- **Type:** Live attenuated vaccine
- **Composition, strain of vaccine:** SA 14 -14- 2 strain

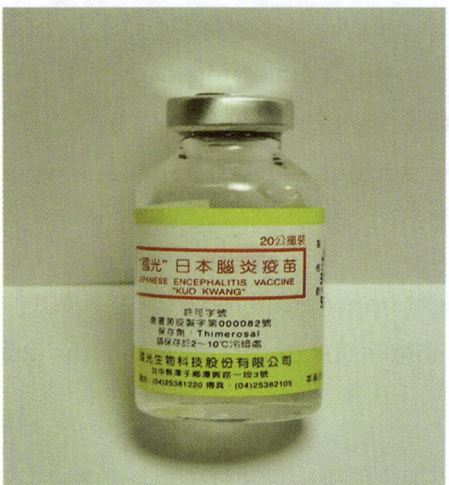

- **Diluent:** Distilled water
- **Adverse effects:** Fever, local reaction
- **Contraindications:** Local reaction, myalgia, fever, irritability, etc.
- **Route and site:** Subcutaneous, upper arm
- **Dosage and schedule:** 0.5 ml , 9 months, 16–24 months [booster](endemic areas)

k. Rotavirus Vaccine

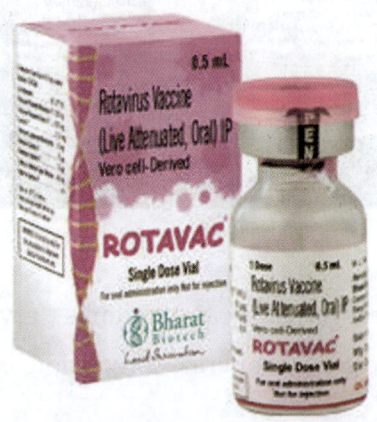

- **Type:** Live attenuated vaccine
- **Composition, strain of vaccine:** Rotavac (ORV 116E) monovalent
- **Adverse effects:** Diarrhea, vomiting, irritability, intussusception (rare)
- **Contraindications:** Immunocompromised state, history of allergic reaction, abdominal surgery and malformation, intussusceptions
- **Route and site:** Oral
- **Dosage and schedule:** 5 drops, 6, 10, 14 weeks

l. Varicella (Chickenpox) Vaccine

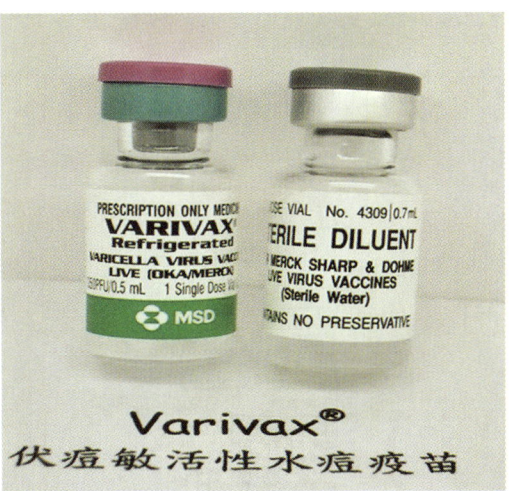

- **Type:** Live attenuated
- **Composition, strain of vaccine:** Oka strain
- **Adverse effects:** Local reaction, fever, local vesicular rash.
- **Contraindications:** Immunocompromised state, pregnant women, allergy to neomycin.
- **Route and site:** Subcutaneous, upper arm
- **Dosage and schedule:** 0.5 ml, 2 dose schedule (4 weeks apart)

m. Influenza Vaccine

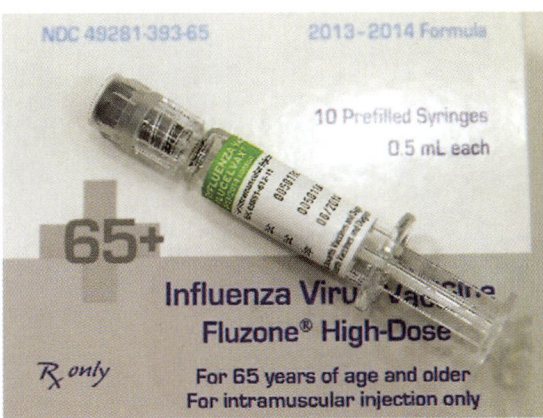

- **Type:** Killed vaccine and live (nasal spray)
- **Composition, strain of vaccine:** Type (A1, A2, B) trivalent
- **Adverse effects:** Local reaction, fever, headache, Guillain-Barré syndrome (rare)
- **Contraindications:** History of allergic reaction and chicken eggs, children less than 6 months.

○ **Route and site:** Intramuscular/subcutaneous, anterolateral aspect of thigh/upper arm

○ **Dosage and schedule:** 0.5 ml, 1 dose (>9 years), 2 dose (<9 years, without pre-exposure)

n. Pneumococcal Vaccine

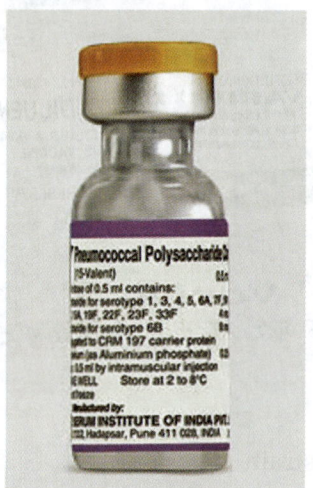

○ **Type:** Killed conjugate vaccine

○ **Composition, strain of vaccine:** Polyvalent (7, 10, 13, 23 valent), PCV 13 used in India.

○ **Adverse effects:** Local site reaction

○ **Contraindications:** History of allergic reaction.

○ **Route and site:** Intramuscular/subcutaneous, anterolateral aspect of thigh/upper arm

○ **Dosage and schedule:** 0.5 ml, 6, 14 weeks, 9 months (booster)

o. Rabies Vaccine

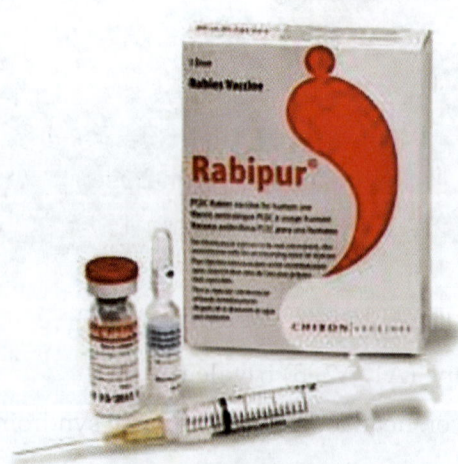

- **Type:** Killed vaccine
- **Composition, strain of vaccine:** Purified chick embryo cell vaccine
- **Route and site:** Intradermal and intramuscular, deltoid/anterolateral aspect of thigh
- **Dosage and schedule—2-site injection:** 0.5 ml intramuscular, 0.1 ml intradermal
  - *Pre-exposure:* Day 0, 7, 21/28
  - *Post-exposure:* 0, 3, 7, 14, 28 , 90 (B) for IM schedule, 0, 3, 7, 28 for ID schedule.
- **Adverse effects:** Local site reaction, fever, headache and GI symptoms
- **Contraindications:** No contraindications for post-exposure prophylaxis as lethal disease

p. Human Papillomavirus (HPV) Vaccine

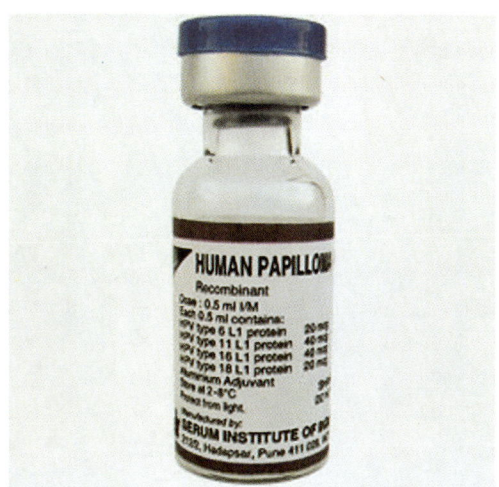

- **Type:** Killed vaccine
- **Composition, strain of vaccine:** HPV (16, 18) Bivalent (in selected states), HPV (6, 11, 16, 18) Quadrivalent
- **Route:** 0.5 ml I/M in deltoid
- **Indication:** Girls 11 or 12 years
- **Dosage and schedule:** 0, 1, 6 months
- **Adverse effects:** Local reaction
- **Contraindications:** History of previous hypersensitivity, pregnant women

q. Typhoid Vaccine

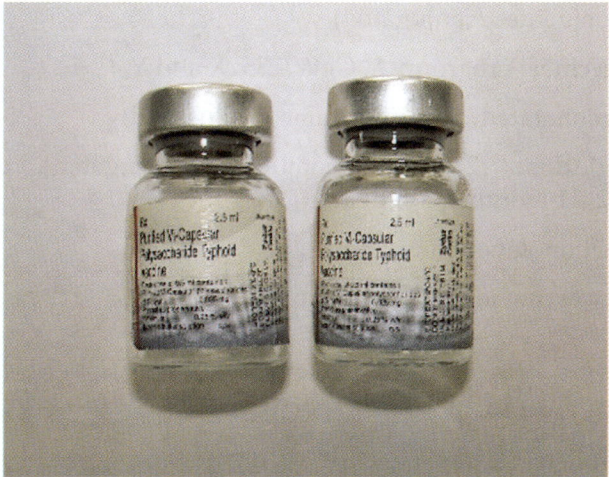

- **Nature of vaccine:** Killed vaccine, oral vaccine
- **Composition, strain of vaccine:** Vi polysaccharide, Ty21a strain (typhoral)
- **Route and site:** Intramuscular and oral, anterolateral aspect of thigh

- **Dosage and schedule:** Given at 2 years (0 doses), repeat booster 3 years for killed vaccine, day 1, 3, 5 oral capsules (for children >5 years)
- **Adverse effects:** Local site reactions (IM), diarrhea (oral)
- **Contraindications:** Congenital or acquired immunodeficiency, acute febrile illness and acute intestinal infection

r. Meningococcal Vaccine

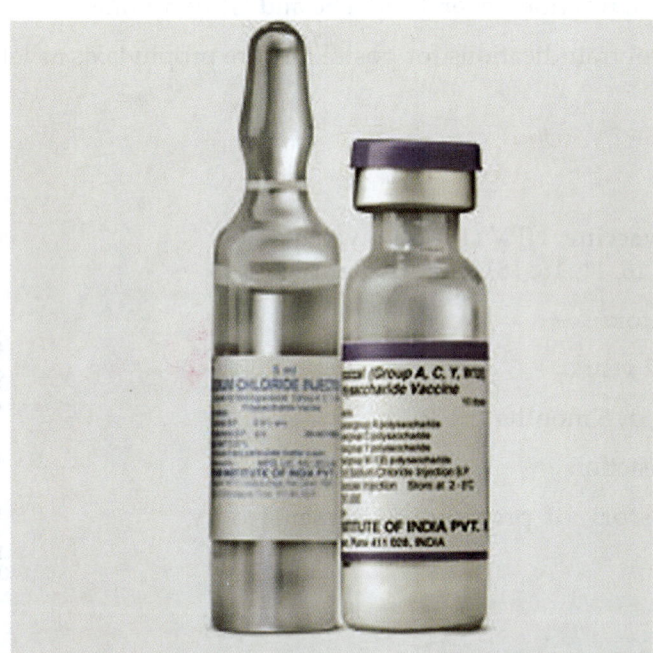

- **Type:** Killed vaccine (unconjugated/conjugated)
- **Composition, strain of vaccine:** Serogroup A, C, W/135, X and Y.
- **Route:** Subcutaneous (unconjugated), intramuscular (conjugated)
- **Dosage and schedule:** Single dose (> 2 years) [unconjugated/conjugated], 2 dose administration 2 months apart and 1 year booster (2–11 months)[conjugated]
- **Adverse effects:** Local reaction, fever
- **Contraindications :** History of previous hypersensitivity, pregnant and breastfeeding women, moderately and severely ill children

EXERCISE

1. Till what age BCG can be given under NIS and why?
2. If an unimmunized infant (11 months) visit health centre, what vaccines will be administered and how?
3. If an unimmunized child (36 months) visit health centre, what vaccines will be administered and how?
4. Apart from routine immunization, what are other special indications for pneumococcal vaccine?
5. Write dosage and indications of rabies immunoglobulin (RIG).

BIBLIOGRAPHY

1. Bharat Biotech International Limited, Genome Valley Shameerpet, Hyderabad 500 078, Telangana, India.
2. Frequently Asked Questions on Immunization (For Health Workers and Other Front-line Functionaries), 2017, John Snow International, Ministry of Health and Family Welfare, Government of India. Accessible from: https://publications.jsi.com/JSIInternet/Inc/Common/_download_pub.cfm?id=19350&lid=3
3. Immunization handbook for Medical Officers reprint 2017, WHO India, Ministry of Health and Family Welfare, Government of India. Accessible from: https://mohfw.gov.in/basicpage/immunization-handbook-medical-officers2017
4. Museum collection, Department of Community Medicine, Geetanjali Medical College and Hospital, Udaipur.
5. Serum Institute of India Pvt. Ltd, 212/2, Hadapsar, Off Soli Poonawalla Road, Pune 411028, India

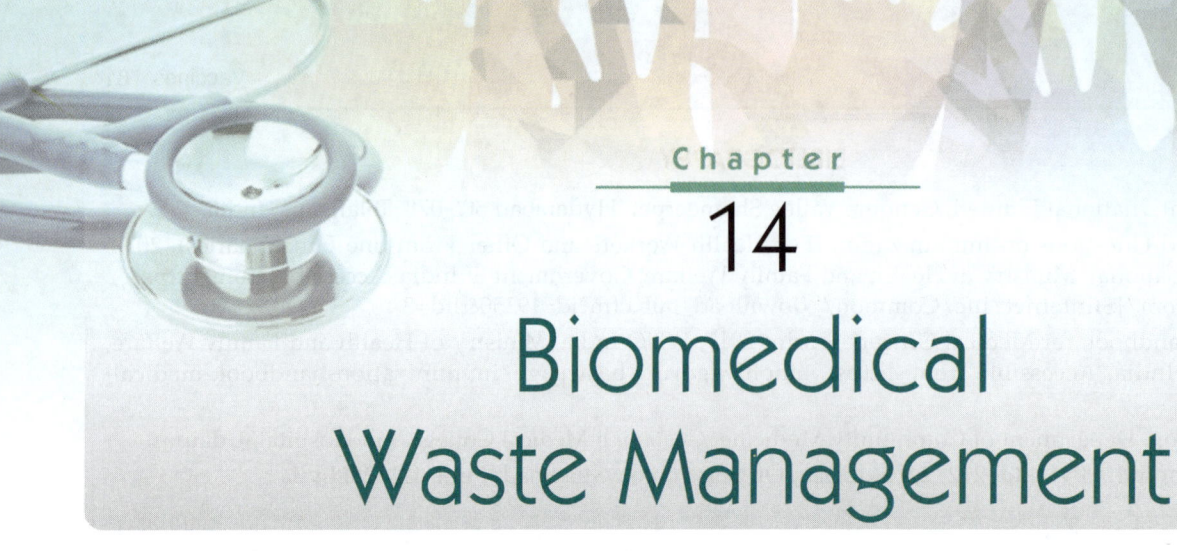

Biomedical Waste Management

Competency		Suggested teaching	Suggested assessment
CM14.1	Define and classify hospital waste	Lecture, small group discussion, visit to hospital	Written/viva voce
CM14.2	Describe various methods of treatment of hospital waste	Lecture, small group discussion, visit to hospital	Written/viva voce
CM14.3	Describe laws related to hospital waste management	Lecture, small group discussion	Written/viva voce

Biomedical Waste

Biomedical waste (BMW) is any waste produced during the diagnosis, treatment, or immunization of human or animal research activities pertaining thereto or in the production or testing of biological or in health camps. It follows the cradle to grave approach, which is characterization, quantification, segregation, storage, transport, and treatment of BMW.

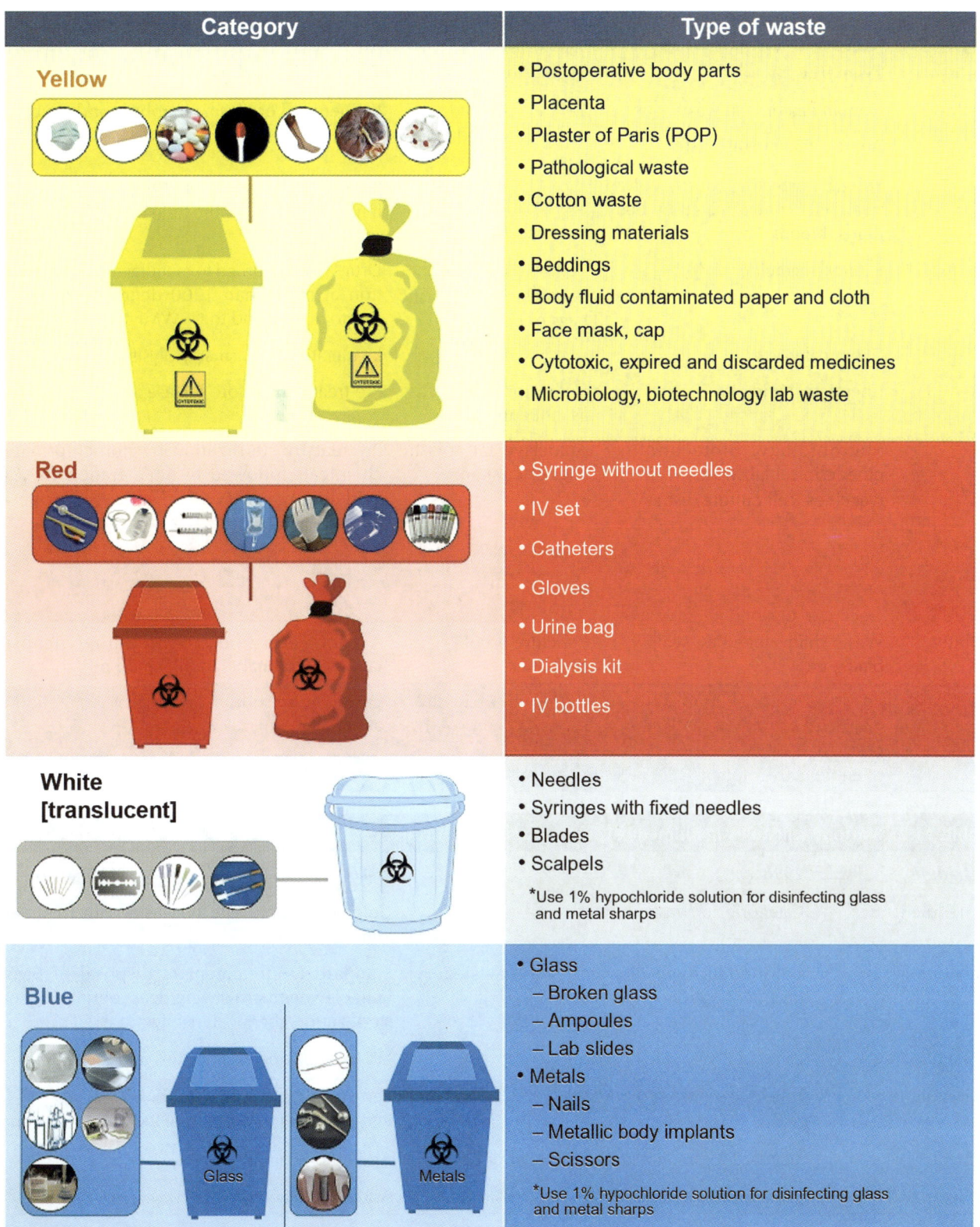

Fig. 14.1: Biomedical waste segregation chart

Table 14.1: Biomedical wastes categories and their segregation, collection, treatment, processing and disposal options

Category	Type of waste	Type of bag/container	Treatment and disposal
Yellow	Human anatomical waste	Yellow coloured non-chlorinated plastic bags or container	Incineration or plasma pyrolysis or deep burial
	Animal anatomical waste		
	Soiled waste (dressings, cotton swab, etc. contaminated by body fluids, blood)		Incineration or plasma pyrolysis or deep burial If not available combination of sterilization and shredding
	Expired medicine	Yellow coloured non-chlorinated plastic bags or container	Drugs to be returned to manufacture or incineration at more than 1200 degree Celsius (for cytotoxic) or send to CBWMF*
	Chemical waste		Incineration or plasma pyrolysis or encapsulation
	Chemical liquid	Collection and release as effluent	Pre-treatment before release as effluent
	Microbiology, biotechnology other clinical lab waste (vaccines, cell culture dishes)	Autoclave safe plastic bags or containers	Pretreat by sterilization by non-chlorinated chemicals followed by incineration (NACO guidelines)
Red	Contaminated waste (recyclable) (tubing, bottles, catheters, urine bags, syringes without needles and gloves)	Red coloured non-chlorinated plastic bags or container	Autoclaving/Microwaving >> Shredding >>Authorised recycler
White	Waste sharps (needles, scalpel, blade, etc.)	Puncture proof container	Autoclave/dry heat>>shredding/encapsulation >>sanitary landfill/sharp pit
Blue	Glassware (broken medicine vials, ampoules except those with cytotoxic waste) Metallic body implants	Cardboard box with blue-colored marking	Disinfection/sodium hypochlorite treatment/autoclaving/microwaving >>recycle

Table 14.2: Various schedules in biomedical waste management rules 1998/2016

Schedule	1998	2016
Schedule I	Categories of waste	Color code and type of waste with treatment and disposal
Schedule II	Color/code, type of waste, waster category, treatment option	Standard for treatment of disposal of BMW (autoclaving/microwaving/deep burial/dry heat sterilization/chemical disinfection)
Schedule III	Label of BMW category/bags	List of prescribed authorities and their duties
Schedule IV	Label for transport of BMW	Part A: Label for container/bag Part B: Label for transport of BMW bag/container
Schedule V	Standard for treatment and disposal of BMW	Added to Schedule II
Schedule VI	List of prescribed authorities and their duties	Added to Schedule III

*CBWMF Common biomedical waste management facility; BMW = Biomedical waste

Biohazard symbol

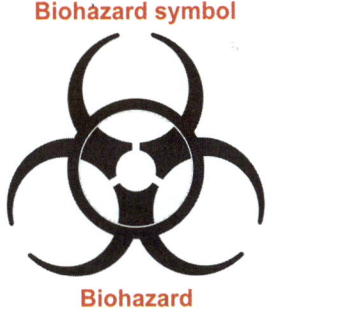

Biohazard

Cytotoxic hazard symbol

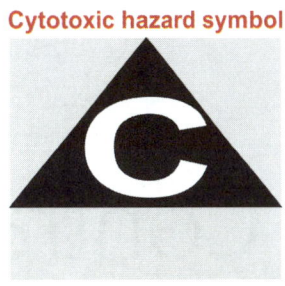

Cytotoxic

Fig. 14.2: Schedule 3, label for biomedical waste containers/bags

EXERCISE

1. How to dispose auto-disable syringes after use?
2. Write the method of disposal of gloves under BMW rules.
3. What is an 'occupier' according to BMW and legal penalties for noncompliance?

BIBLIOGRAPHY

1. Bio-Medical Waste Management Rules, 2016. Published in the Gazette of India, Extraordinary, Part II, Section 3, Sub-Section (i), Government of India, Ministry of Environment, Forest and Climate Change. Notification; New Delhi, the 28th March, 2016.
2. Datta P, Mohi GK, Chander J. Biomedical waste management in India: Critical appraisal. J Lab Physicians. 2018 Jan-Mar;10(1):6–14. doi: 10.4103/JLP.JLP_89_17. PMID: 29403196; PMCID: PMC5784295.
3. The Gazette of India Biomedical Wastes (Management and Handling) Rules, India: Ministry of Environment and Forests, Government of India. Notification Dated 20th July, 1998.

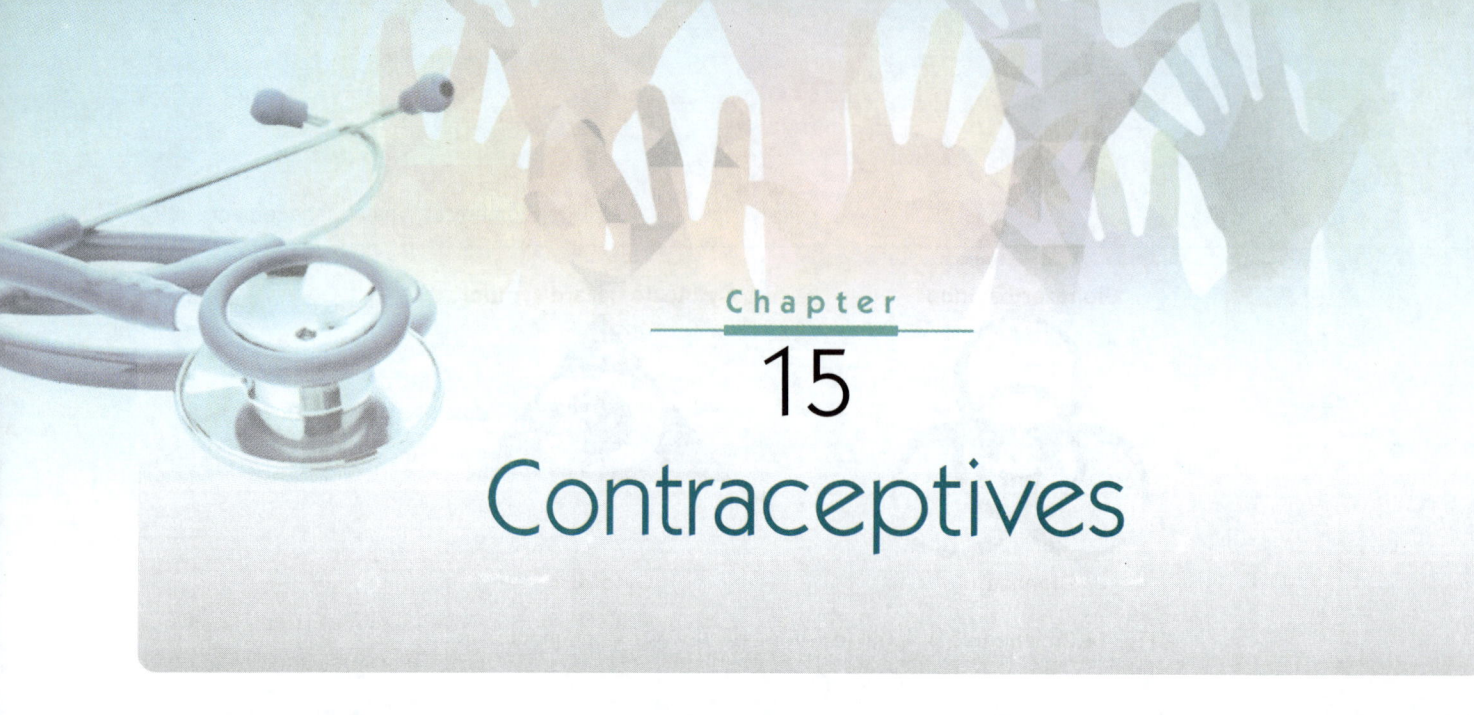

15

Contraceptives

Competency	Suggested teaching	Suggested assessment
OG21.1 Describe and discuss the temporary and permanent methods of contraception, indications, technique and complications; selection of patients, side effects and failure rate including OC, male contraception, emergency contraception and IUCD	Lecture, small group discussions, bedside clinics	Written/viva voce/ skill assessment

A. Barrier Methods

1. Male Condoms

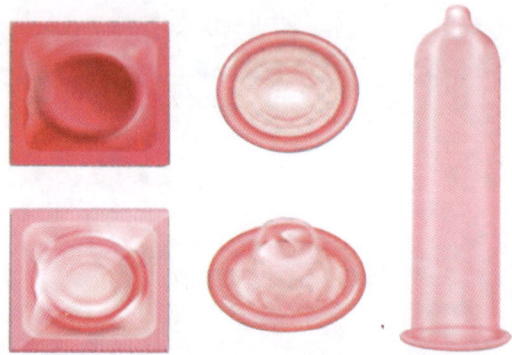

Advantages

○ Protection from STIs, easily available, inexpensive, safe to use

Disadvantages

○ Reduced sensation, may slip off due to incorrect use, latex allergy

○ **Failure rate:** Variable 2–14, >14 HWY (in a few cases)

2. Female Condoms

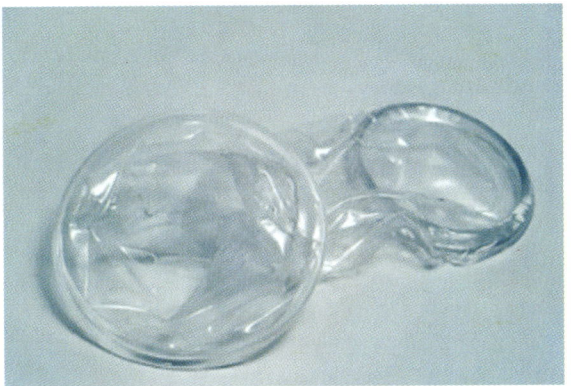

Advantages
- Very few side effects
- Protection from STIs

Disadvantages
- Costly
- High failure rate

Failure rate:
- 5–21 HWY

3. Diaphragm

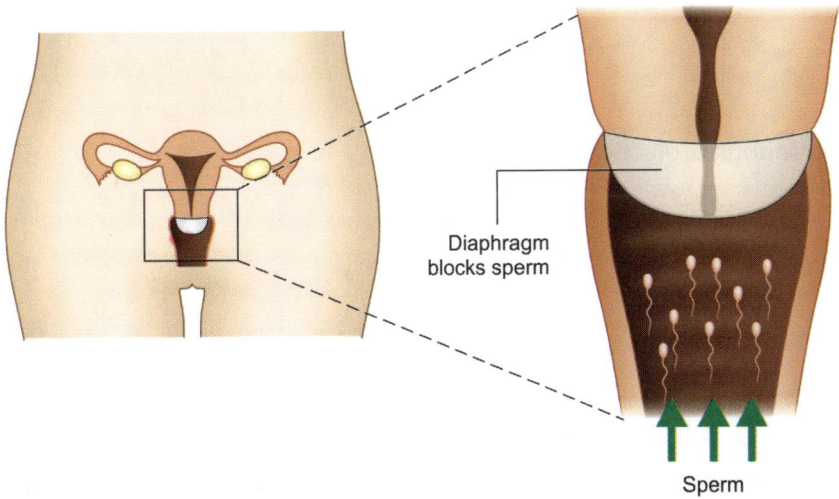

Fig. 15.1: Diaphragm barrier method of birth control

Advantages:

o Safe

o Very few side effects

o Can be inserted up to 6 hrs in advance

Disadvantages

o Not widely available

o Difficult to insert

Failure rate

o 6–12 HWY (with spermicide)

4. Vaginal Sponge

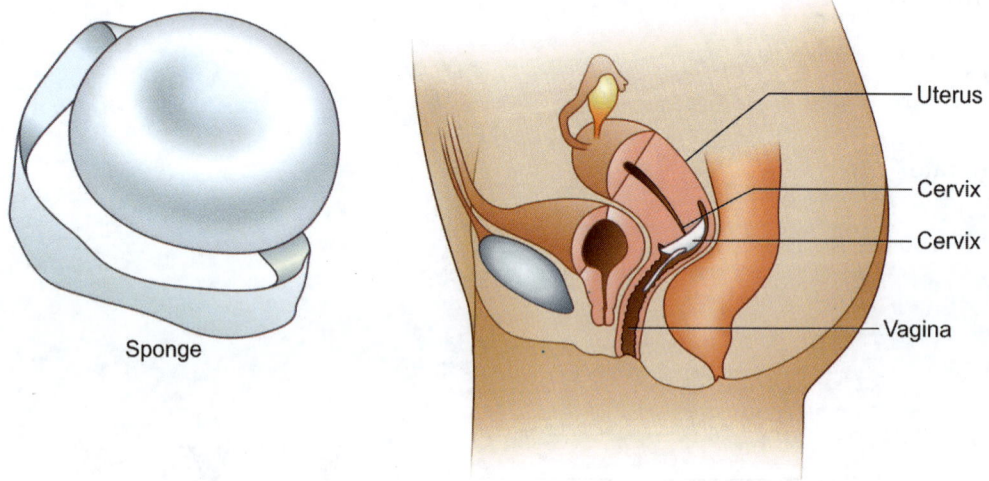

Sponge

Uterus

Cervix

Cervix

Vagina

Advantages

o Immediate and continuous protection for 24 hours

o Easy to insert

Disadvantages

o Less effective

o Removal tricky

Failure rate

o 9–20 (nulliparous)

o 20–40 HWY (parous women)

5. Spermicidal Foams/Jellies/Pessaries

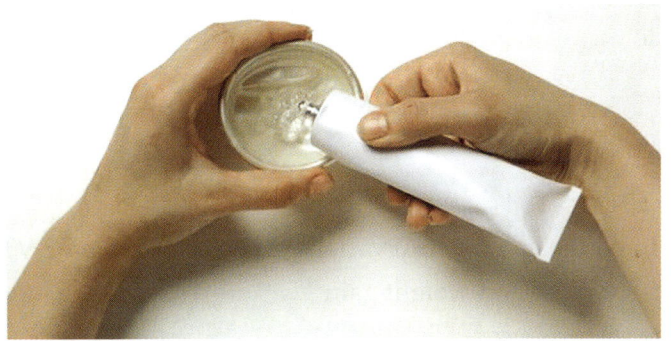

Advantages

- Easy to use

Disadvantages

- Cause burning and irritation
- High failure rate
- To be used repeatedly with each intercourse (pre and post)
- Cannot be used in isolation to be coupled with barrier methods.

Failure rate

- 6–28 HWY

B. Hormonal Methods

1. Oral Contraceptive Pills

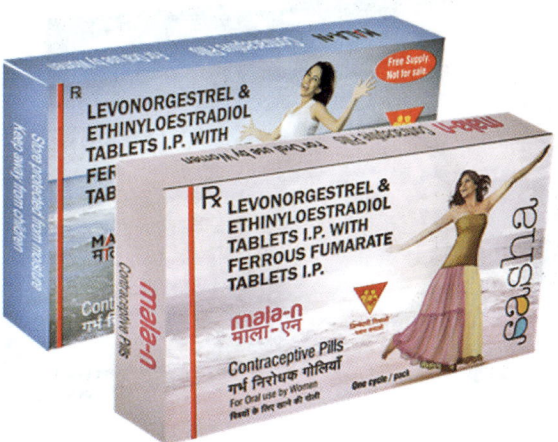

- *Composition:* Levonorgestrel (0.15 mg), ethinyloestradiol (0.03 mg)

Advantages

- High rate of efficacy
- Regulates menstrual cycle
- Convenient

Disadvantages/Side Effects

- Does not protect against STI
- Increased risk of CVDs, hypertension, liver disorder, cervical cancer and DVT, etc.
- Increased risk of breast tenderness and weight gain
- Increased risk of bleeding disturbance.

Failure Rate

- < 1 HWY

Dosage

- Estrogen 0.03 mg, progesterone 0.15 mg

Contraindications

- **Absolute:** Cancer breast, genitals, liver disease, cardiovascular diseases, abnormal uterine bleeding, history of thromboembolism.
- **Relative:** Special conditions requiring medical surveillance (age >40 years), mild hypertension, etc.
- **Non-contraceptive benefits:** Protection against: Benign breast disease, iron deficiency anemia, ovarian cyst, pelvic inflammatory disease, ectopic pregnancy and ovarian cancer.

2. Centchroman Tablets

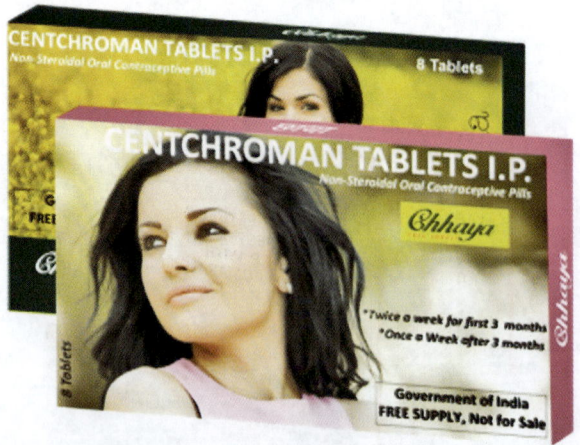

- Brand name of the tablet (introduced by MOHFW): Chayya
- **Composition:** Centchroman (selective estrogen receptor modulator)

Advantages

- Few side effects
- Convenient to take
- Reversible

Disadvantages/Side Effects

- Prolongation of menstrual cycle
- *Failure rate:* 1.8–2.8 HWY

Dosage

- For the first 3 months, 1 tablet (30 mg) twice a week on fixed days
- After 3 months, 1 tablet (30 mg) once a week

Contraindications

- Liver disease
- Chronic illness
- Lactating mother

3. I Pill

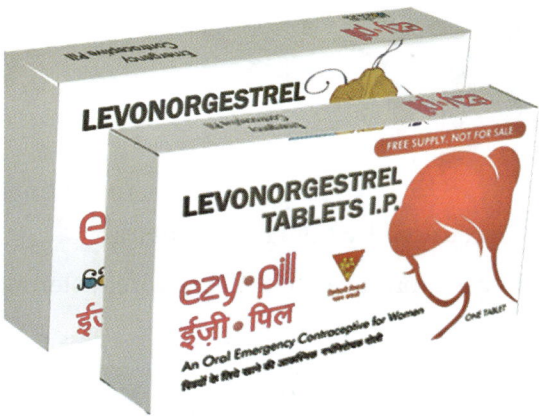

- Brand name of the tablet (introduced by MOHFW): Ezy pill
- **Composition:** Levonorgestrel (1.5 mg)

Advantages

- Single tablet
- Very effective
- Used as emergency contraception (post-exposure)

Disadvantages/Side Effects

- Does not protect from STI
- Most effective within 72 hours of exposure
- Irregular menstrual bleeding, breast tenderness

Failure Rate

- <1 HWY

Dosage

- 1.5 mg single dosage

Contraindications

- Pregnancy
- Liver disease, cardiovascular diseases and bleeding disorders.

4. Injectables

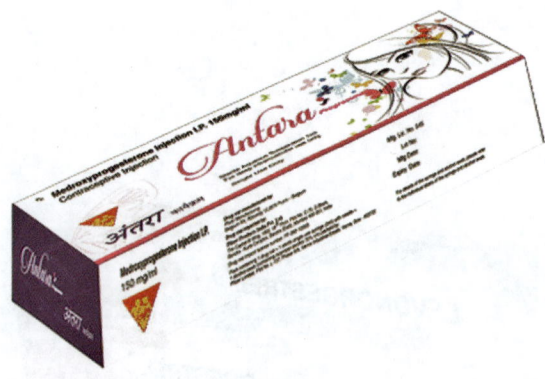

- Brand name of the injectable (introduced by MOHFW): Antara
- *Composition:* Depot medroxyprogesterone acetate (MPA), Norethisterone acetate (NET-EN)

Advantages

- Single injection effective for months (long lasting)
- Safe, effective and high acceptability
- Does not affect lactation

Disadvantages/Side effects

- Does not protect from STI
- Prolonged infertility after use
- Irregular menstrual bleeding
- Weight gain

Failure Rate

○ 1 HWY

Dosage

○ DMPA: 150 mg every 3 months, NET-EN: 200 mg every 2 months

Contraindications

○ Breast cancer and suspected malignancy

○ All genital cancer

○ Undiagnosed uterine bleeding

5. Implants

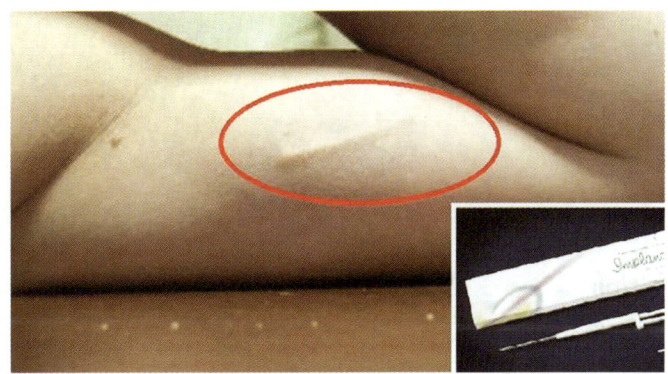

○ **Composition:** Progesterone implant (norplant)

Advantages

○ Effective

○ Long lasting (5 years or more)

○ Reversible

Disadvantages/Side Effects

○ Does not protect from STI

○ Irregularity of menstrual bleeding

○ Surgical insertion and removal

Failure Rate

○ <1 HWY

Dosage

○ **Norplant:** 6 silicon capsules (35 mg levonorgestrel each)

Contraindications

- ○ Breast cancer and suspected malignancy
- ○ All genital cancer
- ○ Undiagnosed uterine bleeding

6. Intrauterine Devices

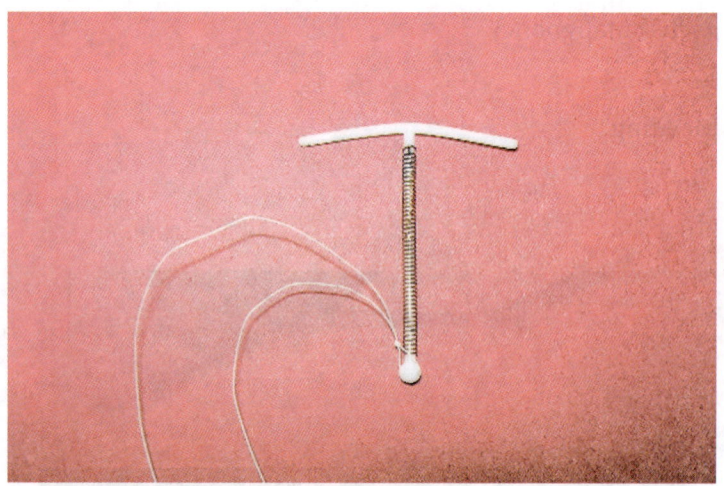

Types of IUCD and Composition

- ○ 1st generation (Lippes loop): Polyethylene
- ○ 2nd generation (Copper T, Nova-T): Metallic copper
- ○ 3rd generation (hormonal, Mirena/Progestasert): Progesterone

Advantages

- ○ Very effective
- ○ Reversible
- ○ Simple and quick insertion
- ○ Inexpensive
- ○ Virtually free of systemic and metabolic side effective
- ○ Can be used as emergency contraception up to 5 days

Disadvantages/Side Effects

- ○ Does not protect from STI
- ○ Vaginal bleeding
- ○ Lower abdominal pain and pelvic inflammatory disease
- ○ Ectopic pregnancy
- ○ Perforation

Failure rate: <1 HWY

Contraindications (Absolute and Relative)

○ **Absolute**

- ◆ Suspected pregnancy
- ◆ Pelvic inflammatory disease
- ◆ Vaginal bleeding of undiagnosed aetiology
- ◆ Genital cancer
- ◆ Previous ectopic pregnancy

○ **Relative**

- ◆ Anemia
- ◆ Menorrhagia
- ◆ History of PID
- ◆ Purulent cervical discharge
- ◆ Unmotivated person

○ **Ideal candidate for IUCD**

- ◆ Who has borne at least one child
- ◆ Has no history of pelvic disease
- ◆ Has normal menstrual periods
- ◆ Is willing to check IUD tail
- ◆ Has access to follow-up and treatment of potential problems, and
- ◆ Is in a monogamous relationship

BIBLIOGRAPHY

1. Contraceptive Updates: Reference manual for doctors. UNPF India, Ministry of Health and Family Welfare, Government of India.
2. Getty Images
3. Importance of family planning, Family planning division. Ministry of Health and Family Welfare, Government of India.
4. Mission Parivar Vikas, National Health Mission, Ministry of Health and Family Welfare, Government of India.
5. My Health Alberta, Govt. of Alberta, USA, accessible from: https://myhealth.alberta.ca/health/AfterCareInformation/pages
6. Park K. Park's textbook of preventive and social medicine. Jabalpur. Banarasidas Bhanot. 2011;463.
7. Shutterstock

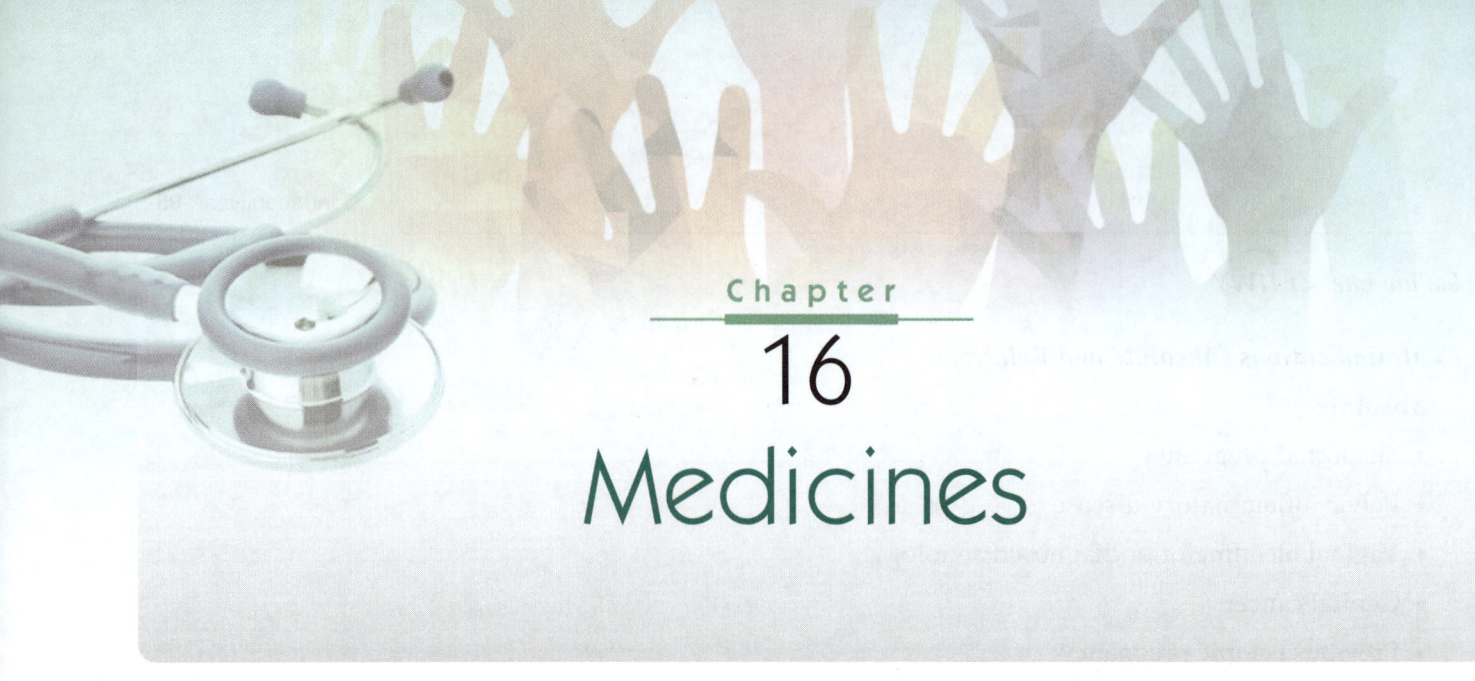

Chapter
16
Medicines

Competency	Suggested teaching	Suggested assessment
PH1.55 Describe and discuss the following national health programmes including tuberculosis, leprosy, malaria, filaria, diarrheal diseases, anemia and nutritional disorders, blindness.	Lecture, small group discussion	Written/viva voce

1. IFA Tablets

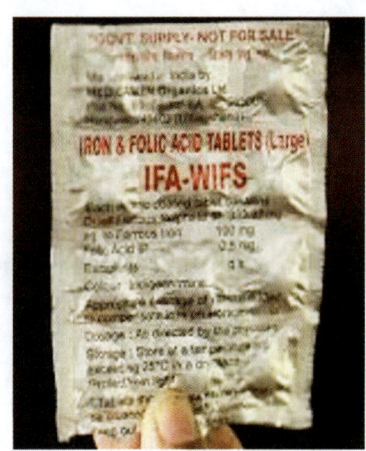

Composition

○ **Ferrous Sulphate:** 60 mg elemental iron (POSHAN abhiyan), 500 mcg folic acid

Dosage

○ **ANC:** 1 tablet daily for 180 days (4th month onwards)
○ **PNC:** 1 tablet daily for 180 days
○ **For adolescents:** 1 tablet weekly (blue colored tablets)
○ **For children:** 6 m–5 yrs (biweekly, 1 ml IFA syrup: 20 mg iron and 100 mcg FA)

       5–9 yrs (weekly, 1 tablet, 45 mg iron and 400 mcg FA) (pink-colored tablets)

2. Oral Rehydration Salt

Composition

○ Sodium chloride (2.5 gm), sodium bicarbonate (2.5 gm), trisodium citrate (2.9 gm), potassium chloride (1.5 gm) and dextrose (13.5 gm).

Action

○ Glucose given orally enhances intestinal absorption of salt and water, correcting the electrolyte and water deficit.

Dosage

○ 1 packet in 1 litre water

Home-based ORS

○ A pinch of salt, 4 teaspoon sugar, 1 litre water

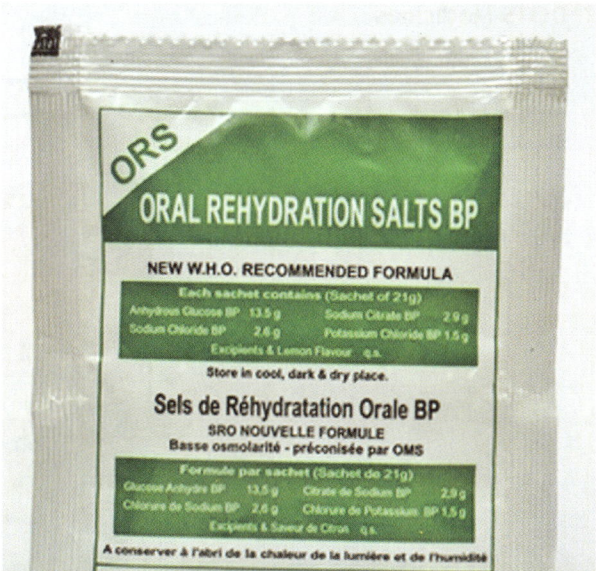

3. Zinc Tablets

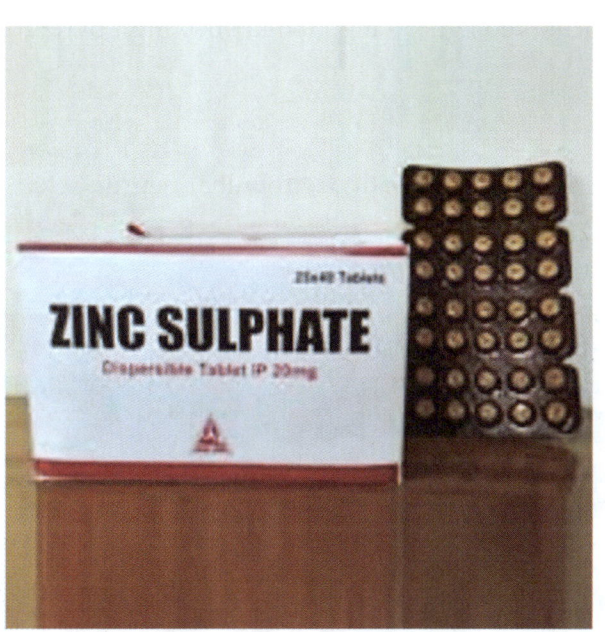

Dosage

○ 2–6 months (10 mg), 6 months–5 yrs (20 mg) for 14 days.

Advantages

○ Boosts immunity, reduces duration, severity and hospital stay in diarrhea

4. DOTS Medicines

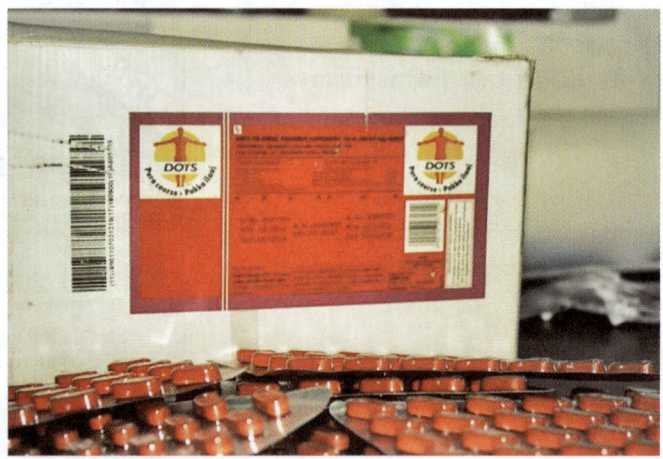

Composition

- Anti-tubercular drugs (first line and second line drugs)

Dosage (Adults)

- Isoniazid (600 mg), rifampicin (<60 kg: 450 mg, >60 kg: 600 mg), pyrizinamide (1500 mg), ethambutol (1200 mg)

Adverse Effects

- Hepatotoxicity, gastritis, peripheral neuropathy, retrobulbar neuritis, etc.

5. MDT for Leprosy

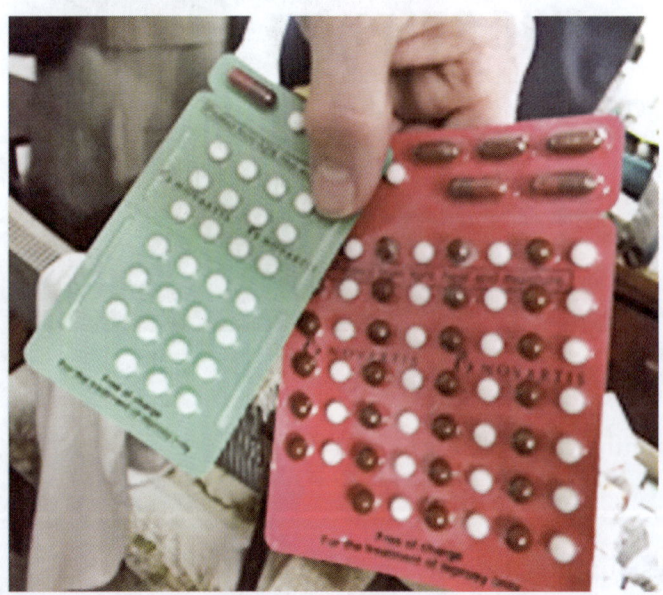

Composition

o Rifampicin, dapsone and clofazimine

Dosage

o **Paucibacillary** [Supervised: Rifampicin 600 mg (monthly), dapsone 100 mg; Unsupervised: Dapsone 100 mg (daily)]

o **Multibacillary** [Supervised: Rifampicin 600 mg (monthly), dapsone 100, clofazimine 300 mg (monthly); Unsupervised: Dapsone 100 (daily), Clofazimine 50 mg (daily)

6. Antimalarial Drugs

Composition and Adult Dosaging

o **Chloroquine** (25 mg/kg divided over 3 days)

o **Primaquine** (Vivax: 0.25 mg/kg for 14 days, falciparum: 0.75 mg/kg on 2nd day)

o **Artemesin-based combination** [ACT SP: Artesunate (4 mg/kg for 3 days) + sulphadoxine (25 mg/kg) + pyrimethamine (1.25 mg/kg) + primaquine: 0.75 mg/kg on 2nd day]

o **In northeastern states:** ACT AL: Artemether (80 mg for 3 days) + lumefantrine (480 mg) + primaquine: 0.75 mg/kg on 2nd day.

o **National Program:** National Vector Borne Disease Control Program (NVBDCP)

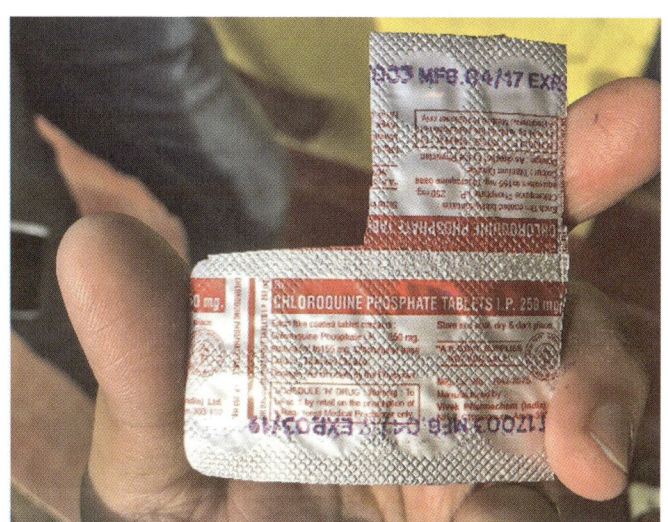

7. Albendazole

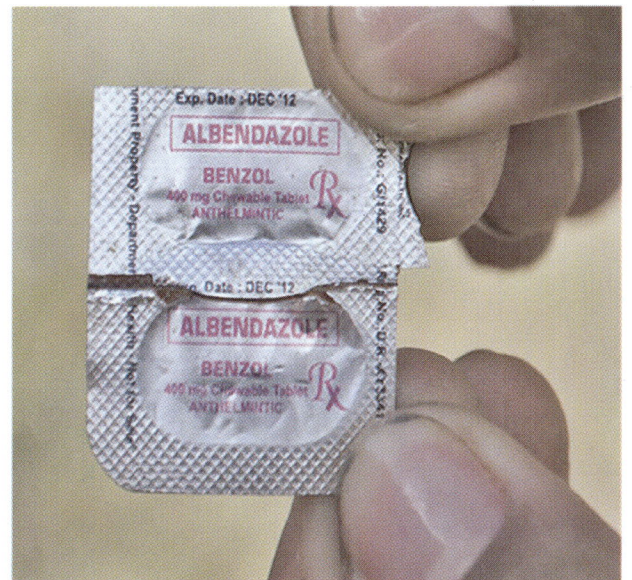

Composition

○ Albendazole

Indications

○ Deworming (ascariasis and filariasis)

Dosage

○ <2 yrs (200 mg) syrup formulation, >2 yrs (400 mg) tablets

8. Rapid Detection Kit (Malaria)

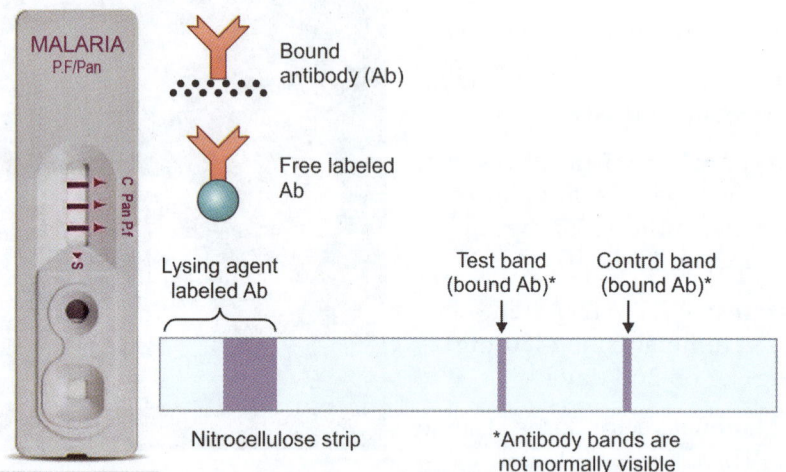

Malaria Types Detected

○ *Plasmodium vivax, Plasmodium falciparum*

Composition

○ Immunochromatographic test for malaria antigen detection: Vivax (lactate dehydrogenase), Falciparum (histidine rich protein 2)

Confirmatory Test

○ Giemsa-stained thick and thin blood smears, PCR test

9. Vitamin A Solution

Formulation

○ Liquid syrup and gelatin capsules.

Route

○ Oral route

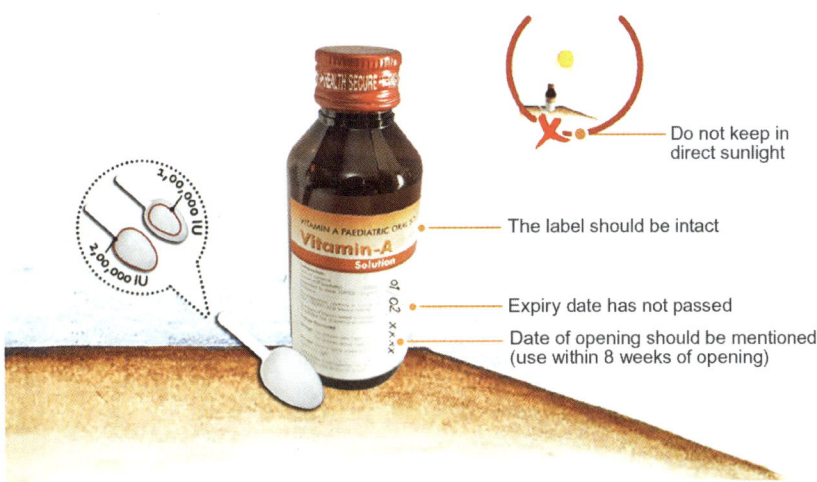

Do not keep in direct sunlight

The label should be intact

Expiry date has not passed

Date of opening should be mentioned (use within 8 weeks of opening)

Dosage and Schedule

○ 9 months, repeat dose 6 monthly till 5 years age [9 doses], 1 lac IU (< 1 year), 2 lac IU (>1 year)

First Clinical Sign of Vitamin A Deficiency

○ Xerophthalmia (dry eye)

First Clinical Symptom of Vitamin A Deficiency

○ Night blindness

10. Kits Used in Syndromic Management of STI/RTIS

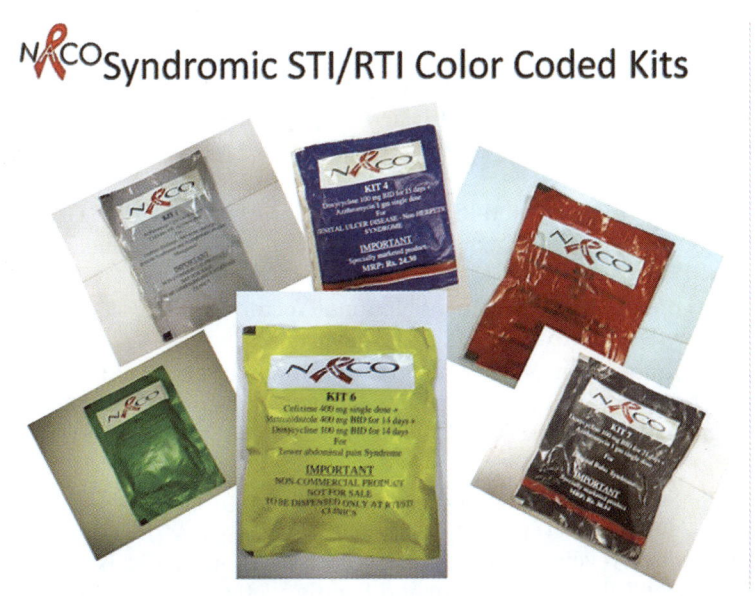

NACO Syndromic STI/RTI Color Coded Kits

Table 16.1 Syndromic case management protocol

Kit no.	Syndrome	Color	Contents
Kit 1	× Urethral discharge (UD), cervical discharge (CD), ano-rectal discharge (ARD) × Painful scrotal swelling (PSS) × Presumptive treatment (PT)	Grey	Tab. azithromycin 1 g (1) and tab. cefixime 400 mg (1)
Kit 2	Vaginal discharge (VD)	Green	Tab. Secnidazole 2 g (1) and tab. fluconazole 150 mg (1)
Kit 3	Genital ulcer disease—non-herpetic (GUD-NH)	White	Inj. benzathine penicillin 2.4 MU(1) and tab. azithromycin 1 g (1) and disposable syringe 10 ml with 21 gauge needle (1) and sterile water 10 ml (1)
Kit 4	Genital ulcer disease—non-herpetic (GUD-NH) for patients allergic to penicillin	Blue	Tab. doxycycline 100 mg (30) and tab. azithromycin 1 g (1)
Kit 5	Genital ulcer disease—herpetic (GUD-H)	Red	Tab. acyclovir 400 mg (21)
Kit 6	Lower abdominal pain (LAP/PID)	Yellow	Tab. cefixime 400 mg (1) and tab. metronidazole 400 mg (28) and cap. doxycycline 100 mg (28)
Kit 7	Inguinal bubo (BIB)	Black	Tab. doxycycline 100 mg (42) and tab. azithromycin 1 g (1)

EXERCISE

1. MDT treatment duration for different categories (color coding).
2. Write the drug dosage and treatment for *Plasmodium vivax*, *falciparum* and mixed infection.
3. RNTCP treatment regimen for different categories (color coding).
4. Write WHO grading of xerophthalmia.
5. What is syndromic approach? How to manage a case of pelvic inflammatory disease according to it?

BIBLIOGRAPHY

1. MoHFW. Government of India. Operational framework weekly iron and folic acid supplementation programme for adolescents. http://www.mohfw.nic.in/NRHM/AH/WIFS/Operational%20framework-%20WIFS/Operational%20 Framework%20WIFS%20MoHFW%202012%20.pdf.
2. National Health Mission GoI. 2015. Intensified Diarrhea Control Fortnight (IDCF). [homepage on the internet]. National Health Mission, Government of India: New Delhi. http://www.nrhm.gov.in/component/content/article. html?id=464.
3. Guidelines for the Diagnosis, Treatment and Prevention of Leprosy. 2018. World Health Organization and National Leprosy Eradication Program, Government of India: New Delhi.http://nlep.nic.in/pdf/WHO%20Guidelines%20 for%20leprosy.pdf
4. Diagnosis and Treatment of Malaria 2013. Dte. of National Vector Borne Disease Control Programme (NVBDCP). Government of India: New Delhi.https://nvbdcp.gov.in/Doc/Diagnosis-Treatment-Malaria-2013.pdf.
5. National AIDS Control Organization, MoHFW, Govt. of India. National guidelines on prevention, management and control of reproductive tract infections including sexually transmitted infections, November 2006. Available at: http://www.naco.gov.in/upload/STI%20RTI%20services/National_Guidelines_on_PMC_of_RTI_Including_ STI%201.pdf.
6. Reproductive, Maternal, Newborn, Child and Adolescent Health program. 2013. National Rural Health Mission. http://www.nhm.gov.in/images/pdf/programmes/rmncha-strategy.pdf
7. National STI/RTI Control and Prevention Programme NACP, Phase-III, India, National AIDS Control Organization, Department of AIDS Control, Ministry of Health and Family Welfare, Government of India.

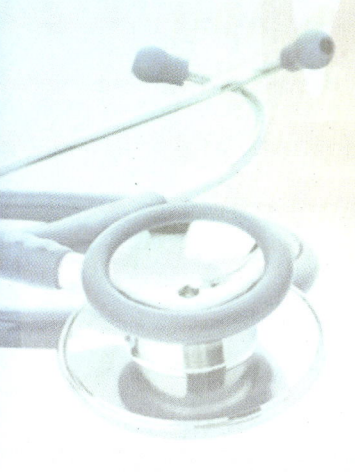

17
Nutrition

Competency		Suggested teaching	Suggested assessment
CM5.1	Describe the common sources of various nutrients and special nutritional requirements according to age, sex, activity, physiological conditions	Lecture, small group discussion	Written/viva voce
CM5.3	Define and describe common nutrition related health disorders (including macro-PEM, micro-iron, Zn, iodine, Vit. A), their control and management	Lecture, small group discussion	Written/viva voce
CM5.8	Describe and discuss the importance and methods of food fortification and effects of additives and adulteration	Lecture, small group discussion	Written/viva voce
BI8.5	Summarize the nutritional importance of commonly used items of food including fruits and vegetables (macromolecules and its importance).	Lecture, small group discussion	Written/viva voce

Recommended Dietary Allowance (RDA) of Indians

Group	Category/Age	Body wt. (kg)	Energy (kcal/d)	Protein (g/d)
Man	Sedentary work		2320	60
	Moderate work	60	2730	
	Heavy work		3490	
Woman	Sedentary work		1900	55
	Moderate work	55	2230	
	Heavy work		2850	
	Pregnant woman		+350	78
	Lactation 0–6 months		+600	74
	6–12 months		+520	68

Contd.

Group	Category/age	Body wt. (kg)	Energy (kcal/d)	Protein (g/d)
Infants	0–6 months	05.4	500	1.16 g/kg/day
	6–12 months	08.4	670	1.69 g/kg/day
Children	1–3 years	12.9	1060	16.7
	4–6 years	18.0	1350	20.1
	7–9 years	25.1	1690	29.5

Recommended Dietary Allowance (RDA)

The average daily dietary nutrient intake level sufficient to meet the nutrient requirement of nearly all (97–98%) healthy individuals in a particular life stage and gender group.

A. Cereals and Millets

1. Rice

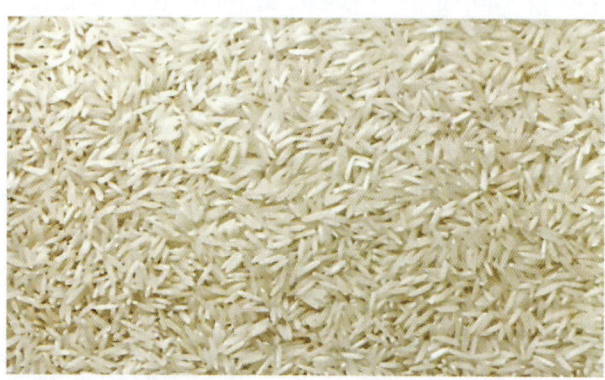

- **Nutritive value:** Calorie: 345 kcal/100 gm
- **Protein:** 7.7 gm% (husked), 6.8 gm% (milled)
- **Limiting amino acids:** Lysine and threonine

2. Wheat

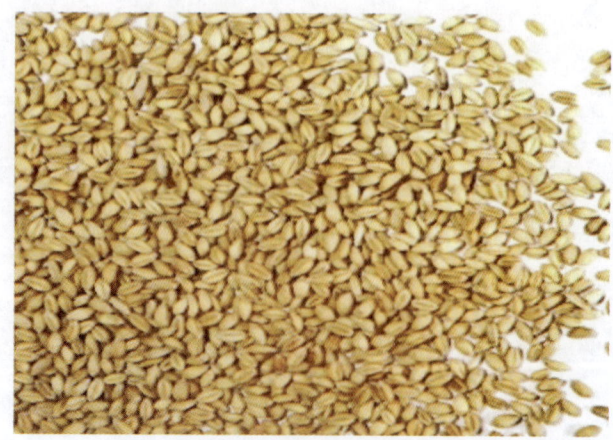

- **Nutritive value:** Calorie: 346 kcal/100 gm; Protein: 11.8 gm% (whole wheat)
- **Limiting amino acids:** Lysine and threonine

3. Maize

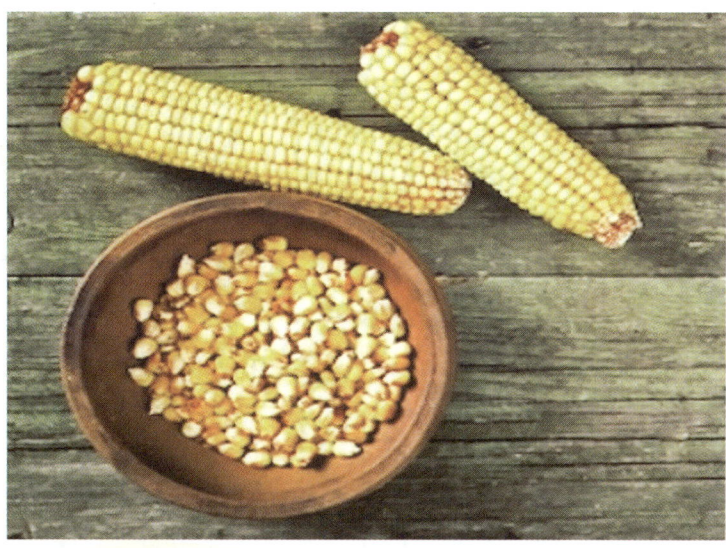

- **Nutritive value:** Calorie: 342 kcal/100 gm; Protein: 11.1 gm%
- **Limiting amino acids:** Lysine and tryptophan

4. Bajra (pearl millet)

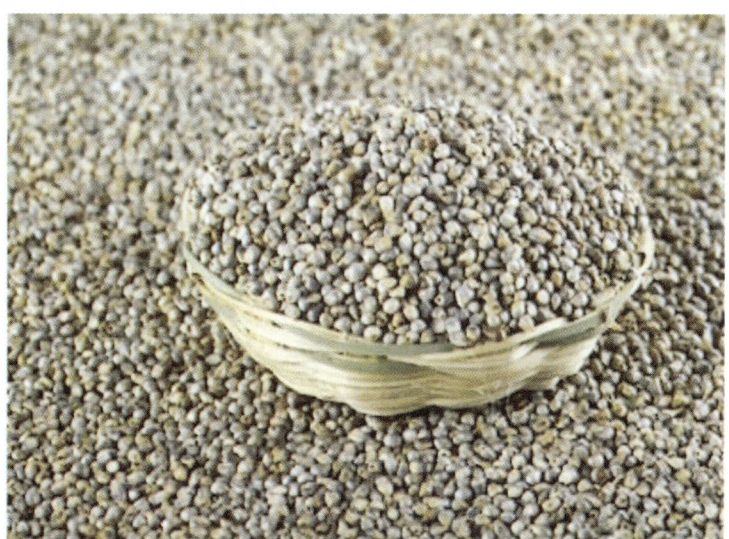

- **Nutritive value:** Calorie: 361 kcal/100 gm; Protein: 11.6 gm%
- **Limiting amino acids:** Lysine and threonine
- **Rich source of:** Calcium, iron and B group vitamins

5. Ragi (millet)

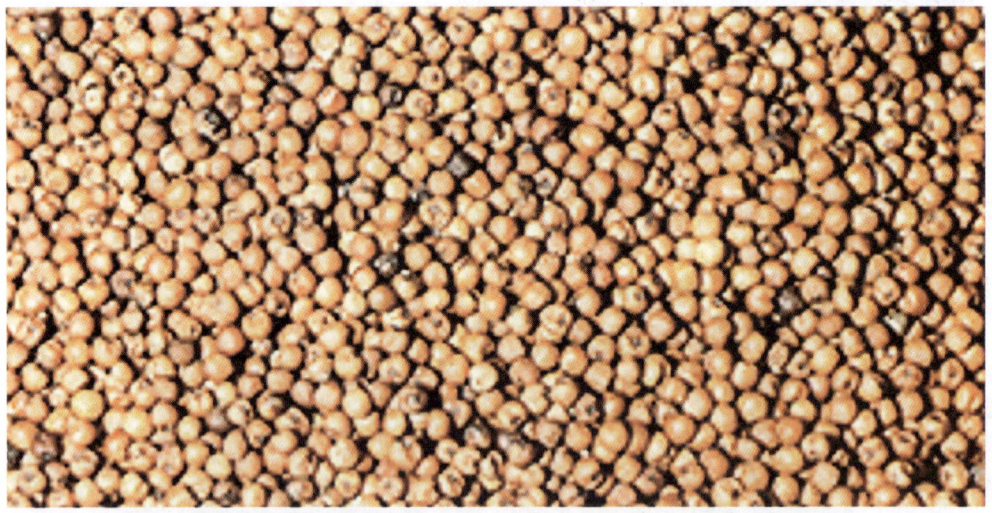

- **Nutritive value:** Calorie: 328 kcal/100 gm; Protein: 7.3 gm%
- **Rich source of:** Calcium

B. Pulses

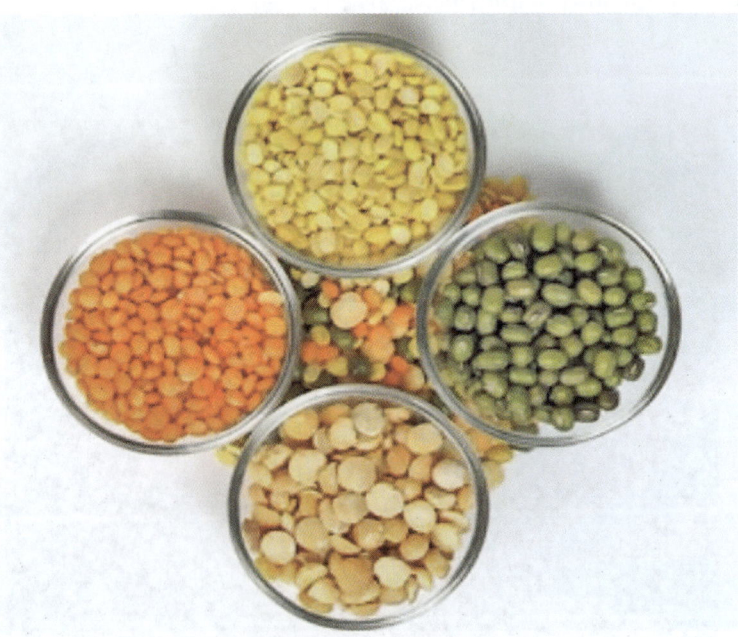

- **Nutritive value:** Calorie: 320–360 kcal; Protein: 20–25 gm%
- **Limiting amino acids:** Methionine and cysteine
- **Percentage of protein content in soya bean:** 40 gm%

C. Nuts

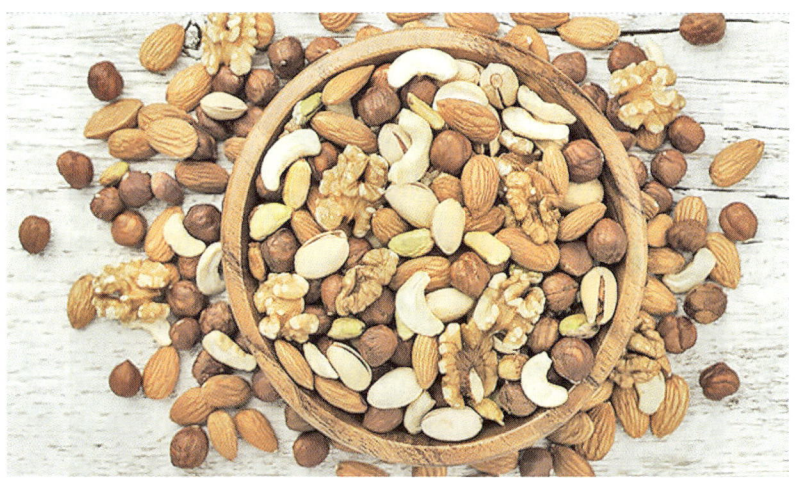

○ **Protein content of Peanut (groundnut):** 27 gm%

○ **Pistachio is rich source of:** Iron

D. Animal Foods

1. Milk

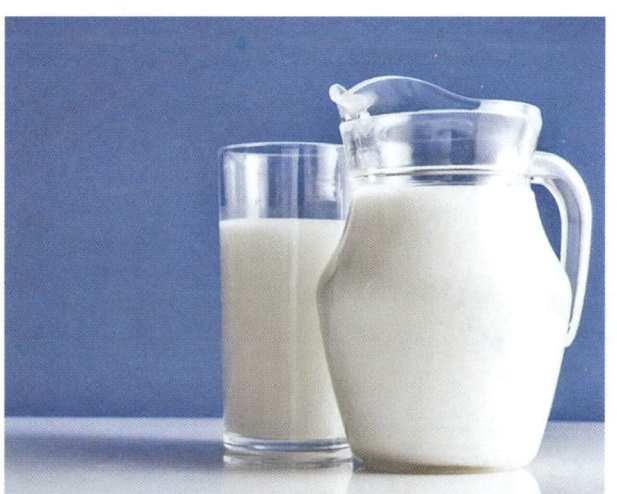

○ **Nutritive value**
  - *Buffalo milk:* Energy 117 kcal/100 ml; Protein 4.3 gm%
  - *Cow milk:* Energy 67 kcal/100 ml; Protein 3.2 gm%
  - *Human milk:* Energy: 65 kcal/100 ml; Protein: 1.1 gm%

○ **Rich source:** Calcium, vitamins

○ **Poor source:** Iron, vitamin C.

2. *Egg*

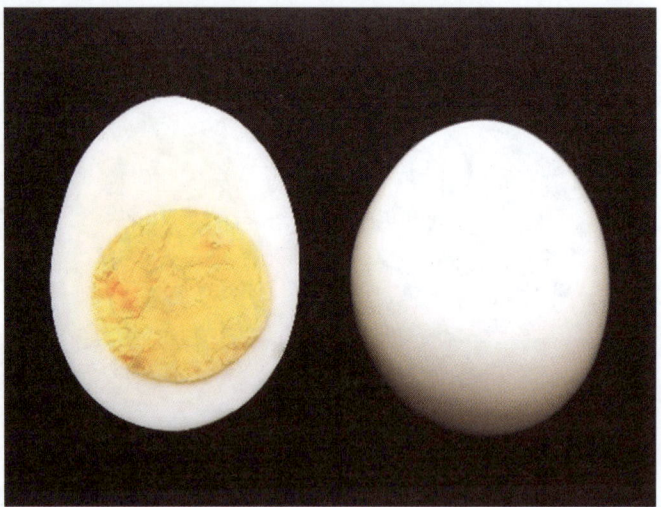

- **Nutritive value:** Energy 70 kcal/60 gm; Protein 6 gm%
- **Net protein utilization (NPU) formula:** Nitrogen retained by body/nitrogen intake * 100 (digestibility coefficient * biological value/ 100)
- Net protein utilization (NPU) of an egg is: 1 (Reference protein)

E. Food Toxicants

1. *Lathyrus sativus*

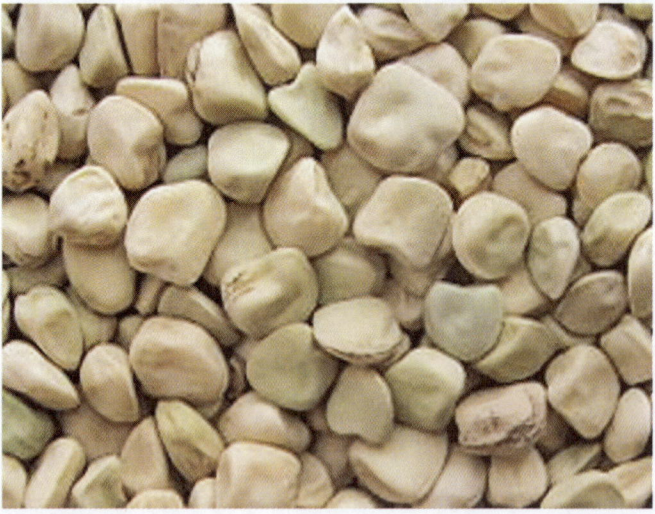

- **Disease caused:** Lathyrism
- **Disease types:** Neurolathyrism and osteolathyrism
- **Toxin:** Beta-oxalyl-amino-alanine (BOAA)

2. *Argemone mexicana*

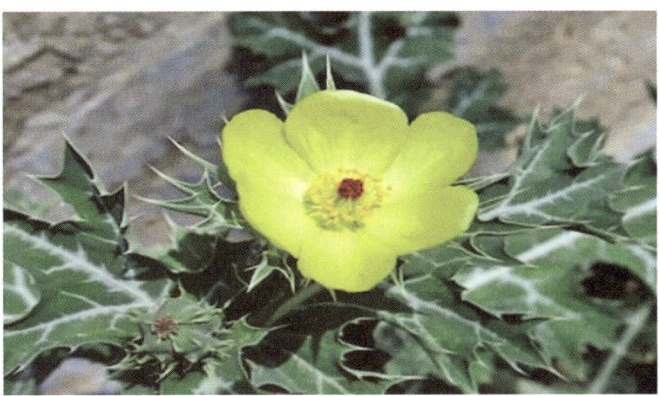

- **Disease caused:** Epidemic dropsy
- **Toxin:** Sanguinarine
- **Tests used for detection of argemone oil:** Nitric acid test, paper chromatography

EXERCISE

1. What is a balanced and prudent diet?
2. What is parboiling?
3. What is complementary action of cereals and proteins?
4. What is pellagra? Describe pellagrogenic action of maize.
5. What are the various indicators for measuring protein quality?

BIBLIOGRAPHY

1. Andrew Butko./ abutko@gmail.com.
2. Das Objekt der Begierde: Reis in rauen Mengen. (Symbolbild) Foto: Shutterstock/matin
3. Dipak Shelare, Stock photos
4. J. Kenji López-Alt, Serious Eats
5. Julia Sudnitskaya/Shutterstock.com
6. Museum, Dept. of Community Medicine, Geetanjali Medical College and Hospital, Udaipur
7. Oqbas/Shutterstock
8. Thamizhpparithi Maari (Own work) [CC BY-SA 3.0 (http://creativecommons.org/licenses/by-sa/3.0)],
9. The Indian fotografo/ Shutterstock.com

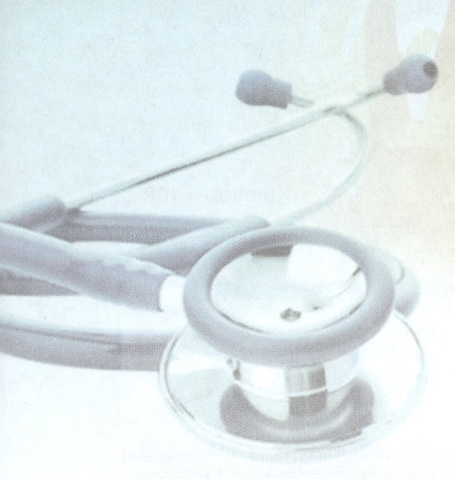

18

Entomology

Competency		Suggested teaching	Suggested assessment
CM3.6	Describe the role of vectors in the causation of diseases. Also discuss National Vector Borne Disease Control Programme.	Lecture, small group discussion	Written/viva voce
CM3.7	Identify and describe the identifying features and life cycles of vectors of public health importance and their control measures.	Lecture, small group discussion, DOAP (Demonstration, Observation, Assistance and Performance) session	Written/viva voce
CM3.8	Describe the mode of action, application cycle of commonly used insecticides and rodenticides.	Lecture, small group discussion	Written/viva voce

Table 18.1   Characteristics of arthropods of medical importance

Vector	Host	Identify	1. Dispersal 2 Distribution 3. Seasonal prevalence	Breeding habit	Resting habit	Longevity
Mosquito						
Anopheles	Domestic animals and man	Head, thorax and abdomen lie in a straight line, wings spotted	1. 3 km 2. Indoor and outdoor 3. Throughout the year, maximum in rainy season	Clean water pond, lakes, river	Hollow trees, bushes, grains and other vegetation	3 weeks, males short-lived
Aedes	Man and animals	Similar to culex, white bend (stripes) on legs and body (tiger mosquito)	1. 100 meters 2. Cattle sheds, poultry farms, bushes 3. In rainy season	Indoor, outdoor artificial clean water collections, tree holes, etc.	Animal premises, green bushy fields	Males (short-lived) 20 days and females 30 days

Contd.

Table 18.1   Characteristics of arthropods of medical importance (*Contd.*)

Vector	Host	Identify	1. Dispersal 2 Distribution 3. Seasonal prevalence	Breeding habit	Resting habit	Longevity
Culex	Man, birds and animals	Head and thorax make angle with abdomen, wings unspotted	1. 11 km. 2. Indoor dark corners, shady places. 3. Throughout the year, maximum in rainy season	Dirty water-ditches, cesspools, sewers, stagnant drains	Dark shady moist places	2 weeks males short-lived
Mansonia	Man	Big black brown mosquito with bands on legs, wings having asymmetrical scales	1. Aquatic vegetation. 2. Throughout year, maximum in summer	Water with aquatic vegetation, e.g. Pistia	Water with aquatic vegetation, e.g. Pistia	8–34 days, males short-lived
Housefly (*Musca domestica*)	Does not bite, transmit diseases	Head, thorax abdomen compound eyes, retractable proboscis, wing one pair, legs—3 pairs	1. 4 miles. 2. Animal and human premises. 3. Throughout year, maximum in summer.	Cow and horse dung (decaying and fermenting) human excreta, kitchen and house refuge	Vertical and hanging objects, dirty foul smelling surface	15–25 days (2–3 wks)
Sandfly (*Phlebotomus species*)	Man and animals	Small (1.5–2.5 mm) light or dark brown colour wings densely clothed with hair	1. 50 yards. 2. Holes and crevices, dark corners, 3. Throughout year.	Damp dark places	Holes and crevices in wall, trees, store room and cattle shade	2 weeks
Louse	Man (*Pediculus capitis, Pediculus corporis and Phthiris pubis*)	Small wingless, blood sucking mouth parts, 9 segmented abdomen	Ecto-parasites of man in scalp, body and pubis			30–50 days
Rat flea (*Xenopsylla cheopis, etc.*)	Rat (specific host), other animals and man also are prone to attack	2.5 mm, bilaterally compressed body, no wings, exoskeleton with bristles directed backwards, blood sucking mouth parts	1. Vertical jumps <6 inches (passive transportation by host) 2. Ectoparasite 3. Throughout year	Rat, burrows and over body of host, storehouse, cracks, crevices, carpet		One month (infected fleas may live for up to 4 years)
Itch mite (*Sarcoptes scabiei*)	Man	Very small (0.4 mm) globular body surface covered with short bristles, suckers present on legs	Ecto-parasites on body of man. Female mite burrows pits in epidermis to lay eggs			1–2 months

Breeding Places of Insects

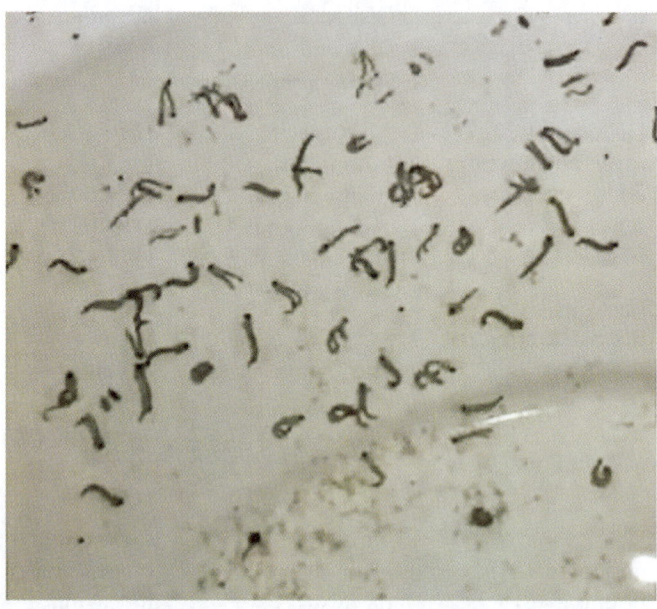

- **Anopheles:** Clean, slow moving water (small streams, fresh water marshes, irrigated lands, etc)
- **Aedes:** Artificial collection water (overhead tanks, coolers, flower pots, etc)
- **Culex:** Dirty and polluted water (open drains, cess pools)
- **Mansonia:** Ponds and lakes with certain aquatic plants
- **Housefly:** Human and animal excreta, garbage, rubbish dumps with organic waste

Anopheles

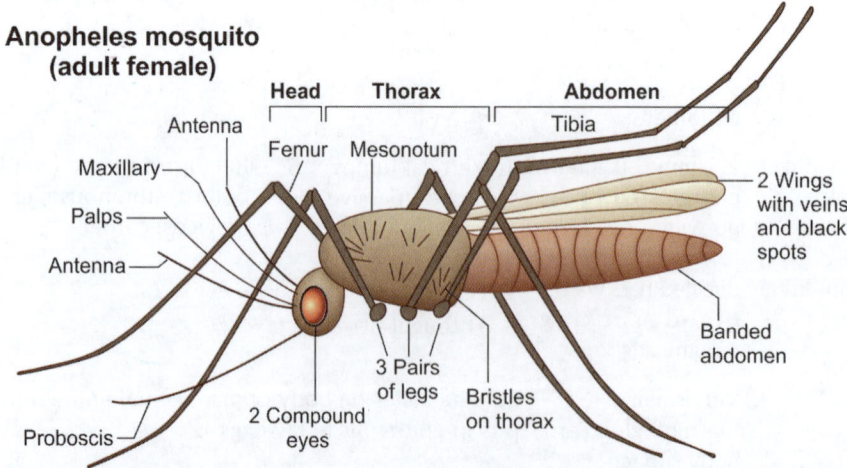

- **Characteristic features:** 3 body parts (head, thorax and abdomen), pair of spotted wings, 3 pairs of legs, inclined at an angle during rest.

○ **Vector species:** Culicifacies, Fluvialis, Minimus, Stephensi, Sundaicus, Phillipensis and Darius.

○ **Vector of diseases:** Malaria.

Aedes

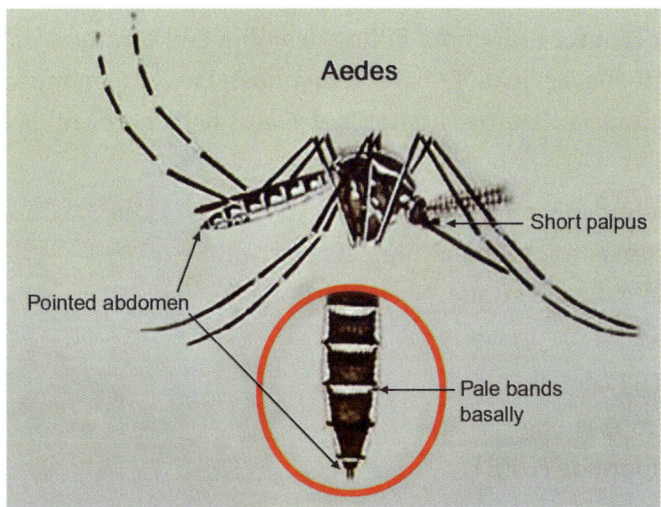

○ **Characteristic features:** 3 body parts (head, thorax and abdomen), white stripes on a black body, pair of unspotted wings, hunchback when at rest

○ **Vector species:** Aegypti, albopictus and vittatus.

○ **Vector of diseases:** Dengue, chikungunya and yellow fever.

Culex

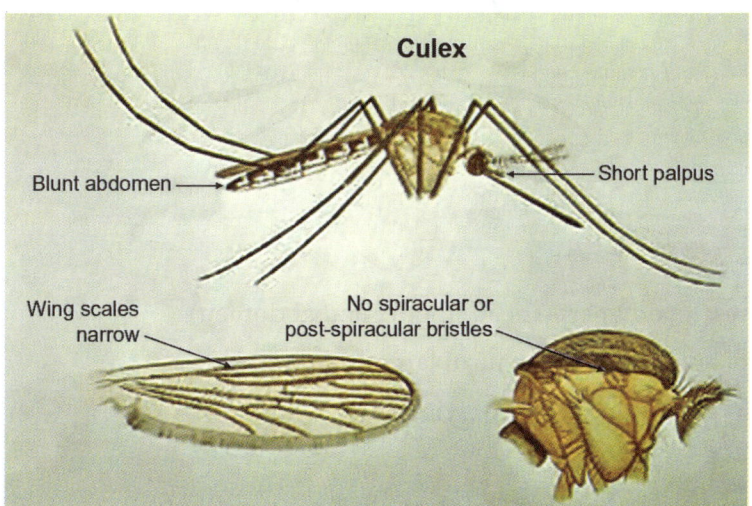

○ **Characteristic features:** 3 body parts (head, thorax and abdomen), pair of unspotted wings, 3 pairs of legs, hunchback when at rest.

- **Vector species:** Vishnui, pseudovishnui and fatigans.
- **Vector of diseases:** Japanese encephalitis, fliariasis, viral arthritis and west Nile fever.

Mosquito Control Measures

1. **Anti-larval measures:**
   - *Environmental control* [Source reduction: Filling, leveling and drainage of breeding places]
   - *Chemical control* [Synthetic larvicide (Abate: Temephos), Paris green mosquito larvicidal oil]
   - *Biological control* [Gambusia/Guppy/*Lebistes reticulatus* fish and bacillus thuringiensis]
2. **Anti-adult measures:**
   - *Residual sprays:* DDT, lindane, malathion, etc.
   - *Space sprays:* Pyrethrum extracts, malathion, etc.
   - *Genetic control:* Sterile male technique, sex distortion, etc.
3. **Personal protection:**
   - *Mosquito nets (LLITN):* Delmethrin
   - *Screening:* Copper/bronze gauge
   - *Repellants:* Diethyltoluamide (DEET)

Housefly

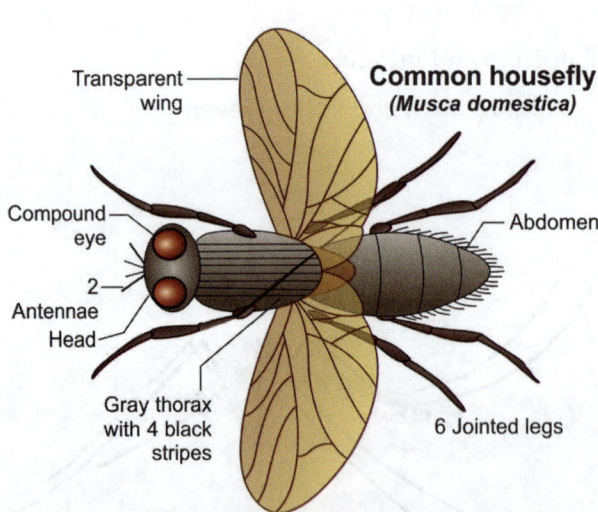

- **Characteristic features:** 3 body parts (head, thorax and abdomen)
  - *Head* bears a pair of antennae and a pair of large compound eyes
  - *Thorax* bears 3 pairs of legs and a pair of wings
  - *Abdomen:* Segmented
- **Vector of diseases:** Typhoid, paratyphoid, diarrhea, dysentery, cholera, polio, etc

- **Control measures:**
    1. *Environmental:* Sanitation and garbage disposal
    2. *Insecticidal:* Residual spray (DDT, lindane and malathion), baits (malathion), cords and ribbons, space sprays (DDT, pyrethrum, etc.), larvicides (diazinon)

Sandfly

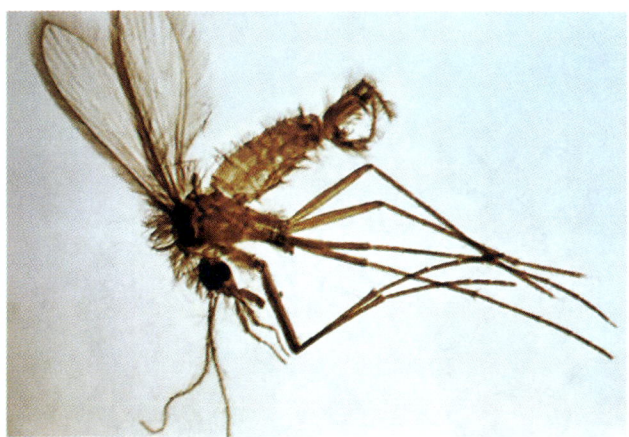

- **Characteristic features:** 3 body parts (head, thorax and abdomen), smaller in size than mosquito, wings upright, hairy antennae
- **Vector species:** *Phlebotomus argentipes*, *P. papatasii*, *P. sergentii*, *Sergentomyia punjabensis*.
- **Diseases transmitted:** Kala azar (*P. argentipes*), sand fly fever, oriental sore
- **Control measures:** Insecticide (DDT or lindane), sanitation (removal of shrubs, filling up cracks and crevices, location away from cattle sheds and poultry house).

Rat flea

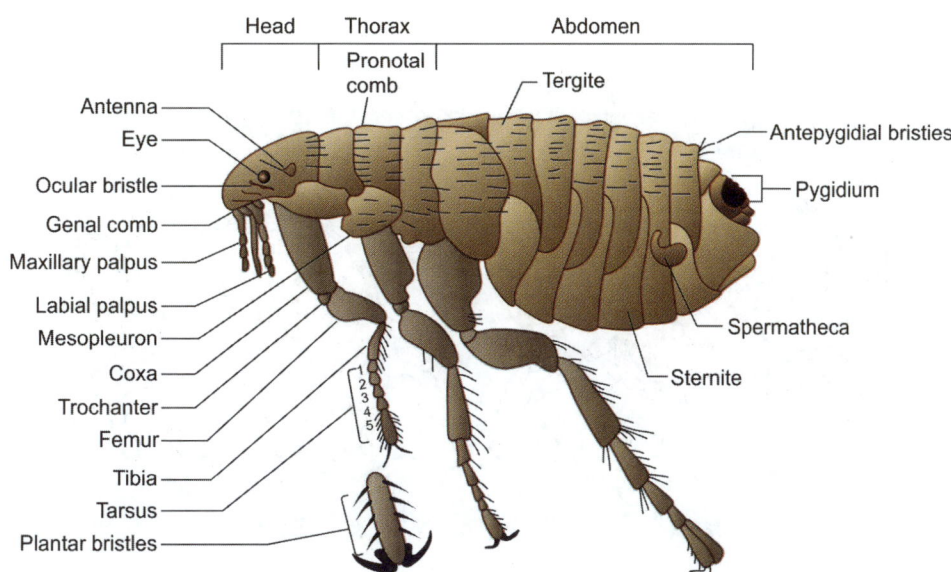

- **Characteristic features:** 3 body parts (head, thorax and abdomen), bilaterally compressed, thorax has 3 pairs of legs, body covered with bristles.
- **Vector species:** *Xenopsylla cheopis*, *X. astia*, *X. braziliensis*
- **Vector of diseases:** Bubonic plague, endemic typhus, chiggerosis and *Hymenolepis diminuta*. (BENCH)
- **Control measures:** Insecticidal (DDT, diazinon, malathion, etc.), flea repellent (DEET) and rodent control.

Louse

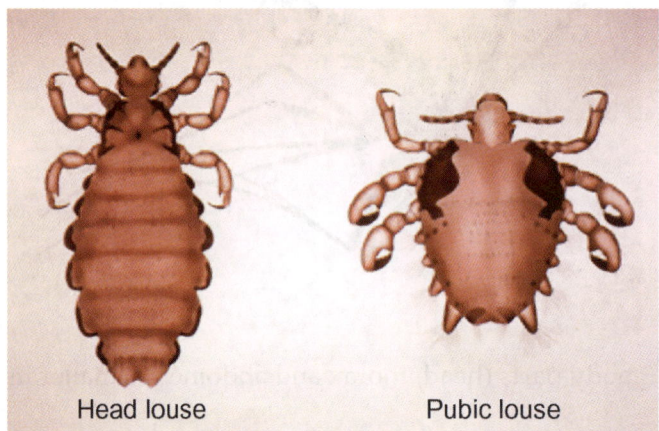

Head louse   Pubic louse

- **Characteristic features:** Wingless ectoparasites, dorsoventrally flattened body, 3 pair of legs attached to thorax, abdomen segmented.
- **Vector species:** *Pediculus capitis* (head louse), *pediculus corporis* (body louse), crab louse (*Pthirus pubis*).
- **Vector of diseases:** Pediculosis, epidemic typhus, relapsing fever and trench fever (PERT).
- **Control measures:** Insecticidal (malathion lotion) and personal hygiene.

Ticks

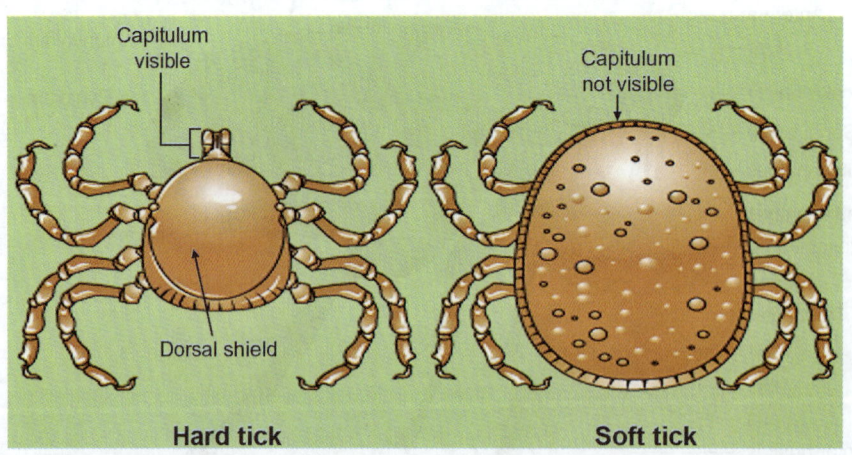

Hard tick   Soft tick

- **Vector species:** Ixodidae (hard), argasidae (soft).
- **Identification features of adult:**
  - *Hard:* Oval body, no clear distinction of head thorax abdomen, head visible from above, four pairs of legs, no antennae, dorsal surface chitinous.
  - *Soft:* Oval body, no clear distinction of head thorax abdomen, head not visible from above, four pairs of legs, no antennae, dorsal surface non-chitinous.
- **Transmission of diseases**
  - *Hard:* Tick typhus, viral hemorrhagic diseases (Kyasanur forest disease), tularemia, tick paralysis and human babesiosis.
  - *Soft:* Q fever, relapsing fever, viral hemorrhagic diseases (Kyasanur forest disease).
- **Control measures:** Animal hygiene, personal protection (insect repellents: dimethyl phthalate), carbaryl, fenthion, propoxur spray

Itch Mite

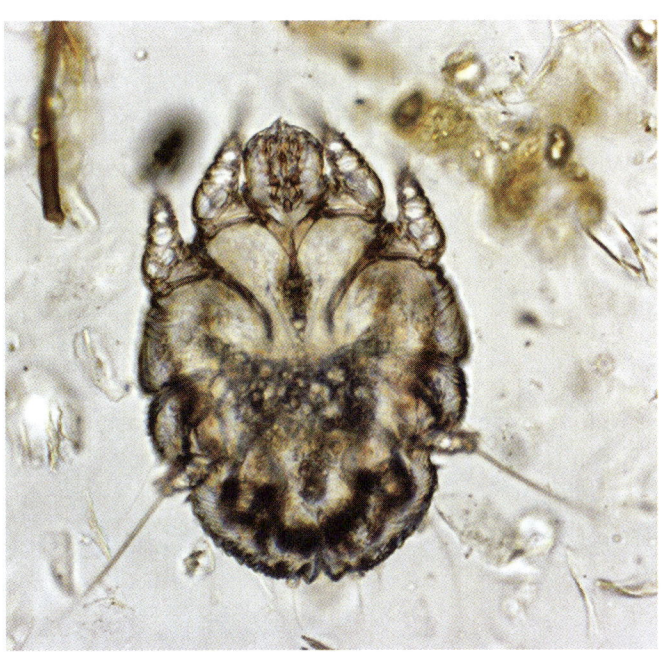

- **Characteristic features:** Globular arthropod (rounded above, flattened below), no demarcation into cephalothorax and abdomen, two pair of legs each in front and behind.
- **Vector species:** Sarcoptes/acarus scabiei
- **Vector of diseases:** Scabies
- **Control measures:** Personal hygiene

EXERCISE

1. Name the indices used in flea surveys.
2. Name the indices used in vector surveillance for *Aedes aegypti*.
3. What are the various epidemiological parameters to assess the burden of malaria in a community?
4. Write the steps in management of scabies.

BIBLIOGRAPHY

1. Park K. Environmental and Health. In Park's Textbook of Preventive and Social Medicine, 25th ed. Jabalpur, India: M/S Banarsidas Bhanot Publishers; 2019.
2. Pictures (Source): https://www.masterspestcontrolsydney.com.au/scabies-mites/

INSECTICIDES

1. **DDT (Dichlorodiphenyltrichloroethane)**
   - *Physical characteristics:* White amorphous powder
   - *Mechanism of action:* Contact poison
   - *Residual action:* Up to 18 months
   - *Repellent action:* Nil
   - *Dose:* 100–200 mg per sq ft

2. **Benzenehexachloride—BHC (HCH/GAMMEXANE)**
   - *Physical characteristics:* White or chocolate colored powder with musty smell
   - *Mechanism of action:* Contact poison
   - *Residual action:* Up to 3 months
   - *Repellent action:* Yes
   - *Dose:* 25–50 mg per sq ft

3. **Malathion**
   - *Physical characteristics:* Yellow or clear brown liquid with unpleasant smell
   - *Mechanism of action:* Contact poison
   - *Residual action:* Up to 3 months
   - *Repellent action:* Yes
   - *Dose:* 100–200 mg per sqft

4. **Paris green**
   - *Physical characteristics:* Emerald green, microcrystalline powder, insoluble in water
   - *Mechanism of action:* Stomach poison
   - *Residual action:* Nil
   - *Repellent action:* Nil
   - *Dose:* 250–500 gm/acre or 1 kg per hectare water surface area

5. **Abate (Temephos)**
   - *Physical characteristics:* Brown viscous liquid and tablets
   - *Mechanism of action:* Mosquito larvicide

- ○ *Residual action:* 25 ml of abate 50% is mixed in 10 litre water and poured in 500 m^2
- ○ *Repellent action:* Yes
- ○ *Dose:* Less than 1 ppm
- ○ *Special features:* Safely used in drinking water sources.

6. **Mosquito larvicidal oil (MLO):**
   - ○ *Physical characteristics:* Oil preparation
   - ○ *Mechanism of action:* Contact poison, suffocate the aquatic stage (larva) of mosquito
   - ○ *Special features:* Injurious to vegetation and fish when improperly used.

Mosquito Nets

The size of the openings in the net should not exceed 0.0475 inch in any diameter. The number of holes in one square inch is usually 150.

Mosquito Repellents

- ○ **Odomos**
  - ◆ *Physical characteristics:* Available as cream
  - ◆ *Content:* DEET (Diethyltoluamide)
  - ◆ *Side effect:* Irritation to skin
  - ◆ *Dose:* 10 mg/cm^2

- ○ **Liquids (All Out)**
  - ◆ *Physical characteristics:* Available as liquid
  - ◆ *Content:* Prallethrin (pyrethroid)
  - ◆ *Residual action:* No
  - ◆ *Repellent action:* Yes
  - ◆ *Dose:* 1.6% w/w liquid

- ○ **Baygon spray**
  - ◆ *Physical characteristics:* Available as spray
  - ◆ *Content:* o-isopropoxyphenyl methylcarbamate
  - ◆ *Residual action:* Yes
  - ◆ *Repellent action:* Yes
  - ◆ *Dose:* 1% oil spray, 13.9% spray concentrate

BIBLIOGRAPHY

1. A.D.A.M., Inc. accessible from: https://medlineplus.gov/ency/article/000838.htm
2. Centre for Disease Control and Prevention. Accessible from: https://www.cdc.gov/parasites/lymphaticfilariasis/gen_info/vectors.html
3. How stuff works, 2007. Accessible from: https://animals.howstuffworks.com/arachnids/tick.htm

4. Museum, Dept. of Community Medicine, Geetanjali Medical College and Hospital, Udaipur.

5. Park K. Environmental and Health. In Park's Textbook of Preventive and Social Medicine, 25th ed. Jabalpur, India. M/S Banarsidas Bhanot Publishers; 2019

6. Public Health Image Library (PHIL). "Labeled Structures of a Flea." Center for Disease Control and Prevention.

7. Tropical Disease Division, World Health Organisation, Geneva, Switzerland.

8. Zoomschool.com

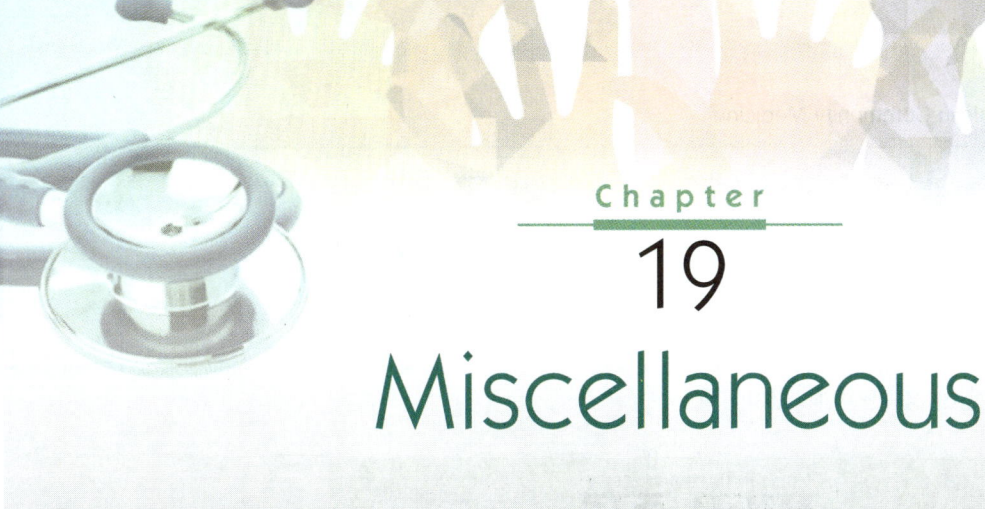

Chapter
19
Miscellaneous

Competency		Suggested teaching	Suggested assessment
CM5.5	Describe the methods of nutritional surveillance, principles of nutritional education and rehabilitation in the context of sociocultural factors.	Lecture, small group discussion	Written/viva voce
CM 5.6	Enumerate and discuss the National Nutrition Policy, important national nutritional programs including the Integrated Child Development Services (ICDS) Scheme, etc	Lecture, small group discussion	Written/viva voce
PE9.2	Describe the tools and methods for assessment and classification of nutritional status of infants, children and adolescents	Lecture, small group discussion	Written/viva voce
CM3.2	Describe concepts of safe and wholesome water, sanitary sources of water, water purification processes, water quality standards.	Lecture, small group discussion	Written/viva voce

MAMTA CARD

Parts of MAMTA card

- Family identification and registration (Janani Suraksha Yojana, Janani Shishu Suraksha Karykram, MCTS)
- Antenatal Care (ANC)
- Intranatal Care
- Postnatal Care (PNC)
- Newborn Care
- Under-five children (infant and young child feeding practice, immunization, etc)

National Program

- RMNCH+A

Uses

- For gaining knowledge related to children's health, nutrition and development
- For using all available services
- For practicing optimal care behaviors
- For monitoring and promoting growth of children.

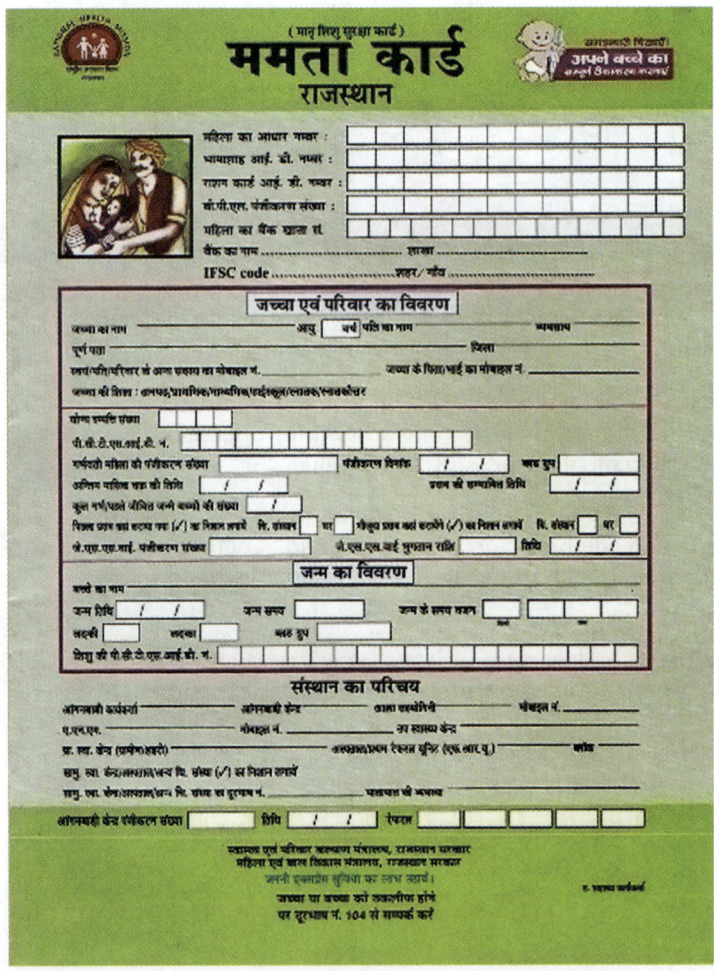

GROWTH CHART

Uses

- Growth monitoring
- Diagnostic tool
- Planning and policy making
- Educational tool
- Tool for action, evaluation and teaching

Parts of Growth Chart

○ Green: Normal

○ Yellow: Below (-2 SD) undernutrition

○ Red: (-3 SD) severe underweight

Detection of Malnutrition using Growth Chart

○ Flattening or falling of child's weight curve

○ It represents growth failure [earliest sign of protein energy malnutrition (PEM)].

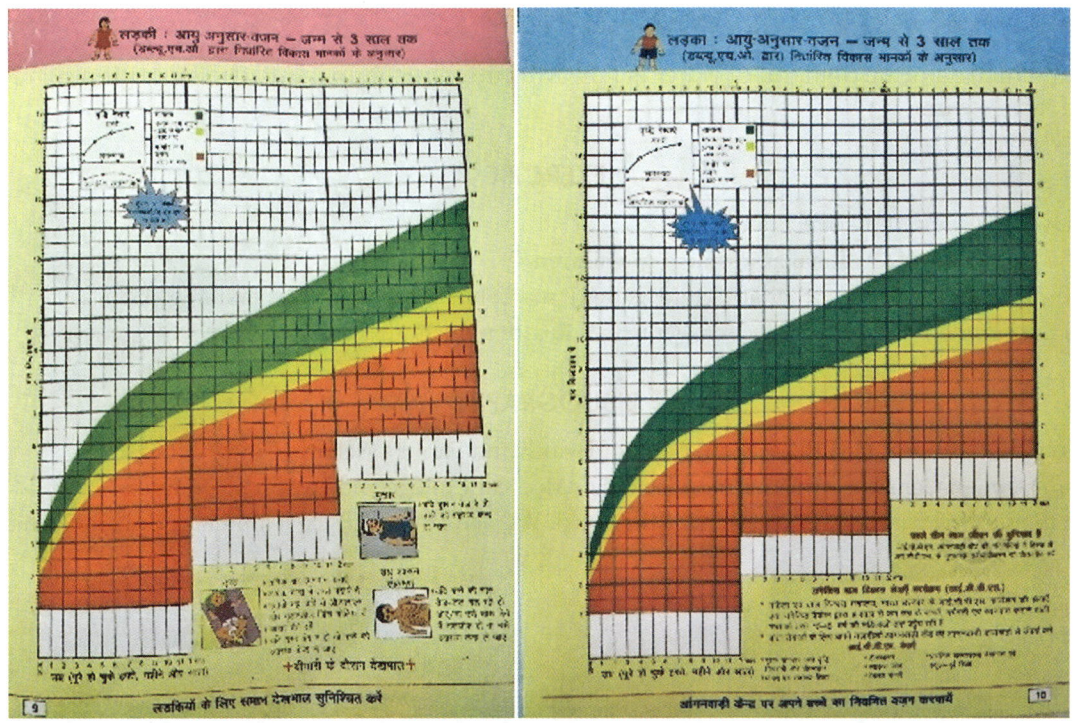

WATER

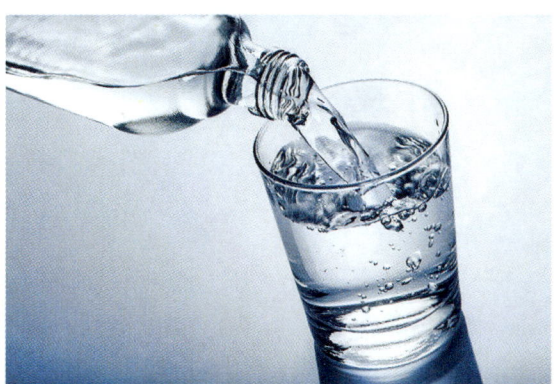

Chlorine Demand of Water

Chlorine demand is the difference between the amount of chlorine added to water or wastewater and the amount of residual chlorine remaining after a given contact time.

Assessment of Chlorine Demand

Horrock's apparatus

Assessment of Chlorine Level in Water

Ortho-toluidine test (OT test)

Break Point Chlorination

The point at which chlorine demand of water is met. Minimum recommended concentration of free chlorine is 0.5 mg/L for 1 hour.

EXERCISE

1. Write down the steps of disinfection of well.
2. Write the methods of nutritional assessment of children.
3. Enlist the benefits given to mother and child under Janani Shishu Suraksha Karyakram (JSSK).
4. What is the criteria for diagnosing severe acute malnutrition in children?

BIBLIOGRAPHY

1. MAMTA Card, National Health Mission, Dept. of Health and Family Welfare, Govt. of Rajasthan.
2. Museum, Dept. of Community Medicine, Geetanjali Medical College and Hospital, Udaipur.
3. Growth monitoring charts, ICDS program, Ministry of Women and Child Development, Govt. of India.

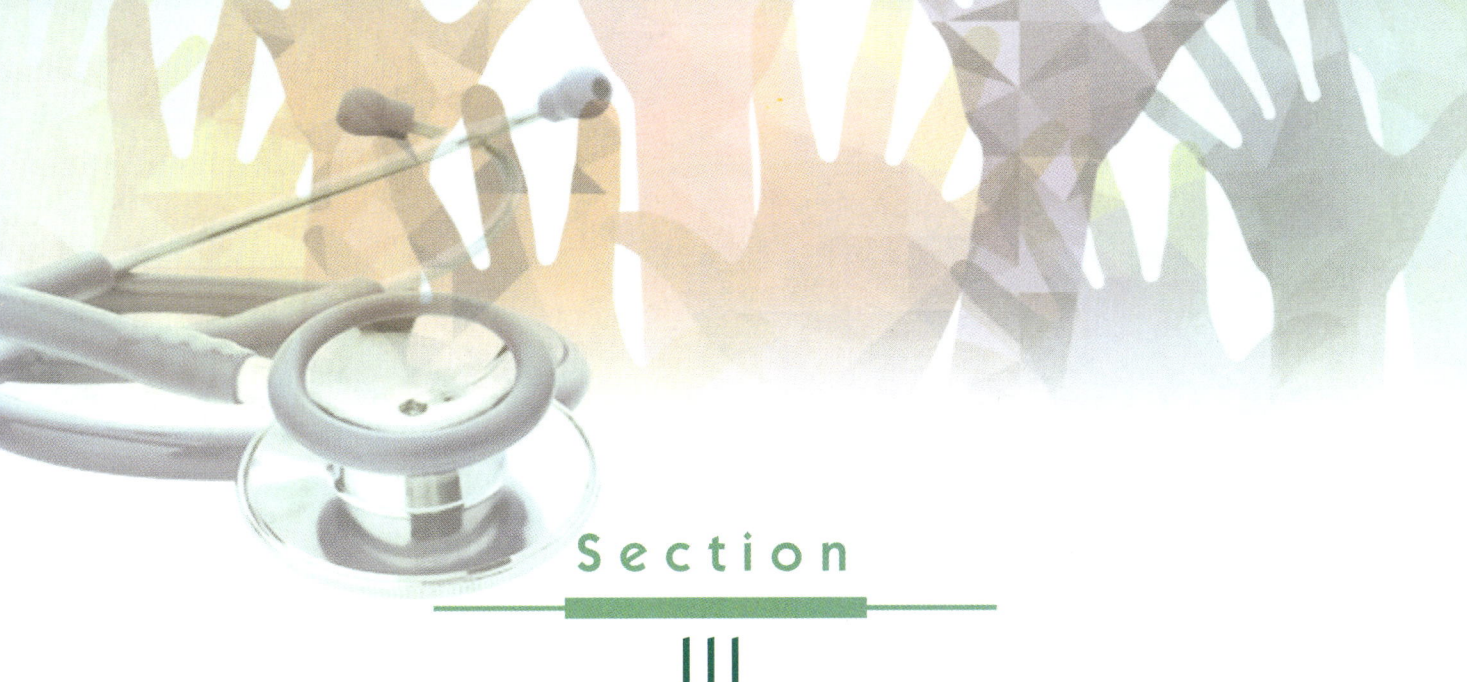

Epidemiological and Statistical Exercises

- Fertility-based Indicators
- Data and its Presentation
- Measures of Central Tendency and Dispersion
- Tests of Significance
- Screening Test
- Investigation of an Outbreak

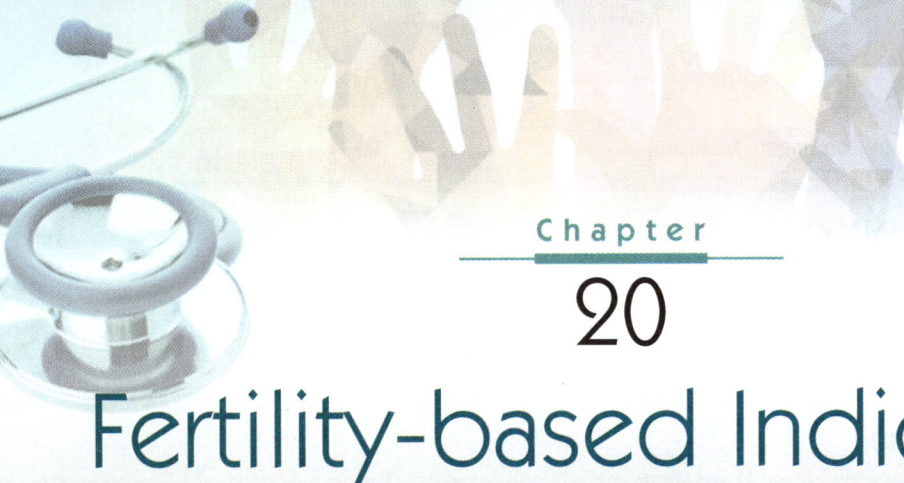

20

Fertility-based Indicators

Competency		Suggested teaching	Suggested assessment
CM9.1	Define and describe the principles of demography, demographic cycle, vital statistics	Small group discussion, lecture	Written/viva voce
CM9.2	Define, calculate and interpret demographic indices including birth rate, death rate, fertility rates	Lecture, small group discussion, DOAP (Demonstration, Observation, Assistance and Performance) sessions	Skill assessment

A. Demographic Indices

1. **Birth Rate (BR):** Simplest indicator of fertility

$$BR = \frac{\text{Number of live births during the year}}{\text{Estimated mid-year population}} \times 1000$$

2. **General Fertility Rate (GFR)**

$$GFR = \frac{\text{Number of live births during the year}}{\text{Mid-year female population (15 – 44 yrs)}} \times 1000$$

3. **Age Specific Fertility Rate (ASFR):**

$$ASFR = \frac{\text{Number of live births in a particular age group}}{\text{Mid-year female population of same age group}} \times 1000$$

4. **Total Fertility Rate:** It represents the average number of children a woman would have if she were to pass through her reproductive years bearing children at the same rates as the women now in each group

5. **Gross Reproduction Rate:** Average number of girls that would be born to a woman if she experiences the current fertility pattern throughout her reproductive span (15–44 or 49 years), assuming no mortality.

6. **Net Reproduction Rate (NRR):** Number of daughters a newborn girl will bear during her lifetime assuming fixed age-specific fertility and mortality rates.

NRR is a demographic indicator. NRR of 1 is equivalent to attaining approximately the 2 child norm.

7. **Maternal Mortality Ratio (MMR):**

$$MMR = \frac{\text{Total no. of female deaths due to complications of pregnancy, childbirth Or within 42 days of delivery from puerperal causes in a year}}{\text{Total no. of live births in the same area and year}} \times 100{,}000$$

8. **Infant Mortality Rate (IMR):**

$$IMR = \frac{\text{Number of child deaths under one year of age}}{\text{Total no. of live births}} \times 1000$$

9. **Under-5 Mortality Rate:**

$$\text{U-5 MR} = \frac{\text{Number of child deaths under five years of age}}{\text{Total no. of live births}} \times 1000$$

10. **Couple Protection Rate (CPR):** It is an indicator of the prevalence of contraceptive practice in the community.

$$CPR = \frac{\text{Eligible couples using contraception}}{\text{Total no. of eligible couples}} \times 100$$

11. **Pearl index:** It is defined as the number of failures per 100 woman years (HWY) of exposure

$$\text{Failure rate per HWY} = \frac{\text{Total accidental pregnancies}}{\text{Total months of exposure}} \times 1200$$

B. Exercise

1. **Calculate the total fertility rate and gross reproduction rate (sex ratio 1:1) from the following data for a particular year.**

Age group	No. of women in the age group	No. of live births in the age group
15–19	250	12
20–24	450	95
25–29	425	75
30–34	400	40
35–39	240	15
40–44	200	5

Ans.   TFR represents the average number of children a woman would have if she were to pass through her reproductive years bearing children at the same rates as the women now in each group.

After calculating ASFR,

$$\text{Total fertility rate} = \frac{5 \times \Sigma\left(\text{ASFR}_{15-19} \text{ to ASFR}_{45-49}\right)}{1000}$$

Age-specific fertility rate has been calculated by using the formula:

$$\text{ASFR} = \frac{\text{No. of live births in a particular age group}}{\text{Mid-year female population of the same age group}} \times 1000$$

$\text{ASFR}_{15-19} = 12/250 \times 1000 = 48$

$\text{ASFR}_{20-24} = 95/450 \times 1000 = 211$

$\text{ASFR}_{25-29} = 75/425 \times 1000 = 176$

$\text{ASFR}_{30-34} = 40/400 \times 1000 = 100$

$\text{ASFR}_{35-39} = 15/240 \times 1000 = 62.5$

$\text{ASFR}_{40-44} = 5/200 \times 1000 = 25$

After calculating ASFR for each group,

$$\text{TRR} = \frac{5 \times \Sigma\left(\text{ASFR}_{15-19} \text{ to ASFR}_{45-49}\right)}{1000}$$

$$\text{TRR} = \frac{5 \times (48 + 211 + 176 + 100 + 62.5 + 25)}{1000} = 3.1$$

$$\text{GRR} = \frac{5 \times \Sigma(\text{ASFR for female births})}{1000}$$

$$\text{GRR} = \frac{5 \times \Sigma(\text{ASFR}_{15-19} \text{ to ASFR}_{45-49}) \times \frac{1}{2} \text{ (since sex ratio is given to be 1:1)}}{1000}$$

$$= \frac{5 \times (622.5/2)}{1000} = 1.56$$

2. **A community has a population of 30,000 and a birth rate of 36 per 1000. 5 maternal deaths were reported in the current year. Calculate the MMR.**

Ans.

Total live births: $36 \times 30 = 1080$

Using the formula =

$$\text{Maternal mortality ratio} = \frac{\substack{\text{Total no. of deaths due to complications of pregnancy,} \\ \text{childbirth or within 42 days of delivery from} \\ \text{puerperal causes in an area during a given year}}}{\text{Total no. of live births in the same area and year}} \times 100000 \text{ (lac)}$$

$$MMR = \frac{5 \times 100000}{1080}$$

MMR = 462/lac live births

3. **A contraceptive is used by 100 couples for a continuous period of 2 years. During this period 20 women become pregnant despite using contraceptive. Calculate the pearl index of this contraceptive.**

Ans.

$$Pearl\ index = \frac{Total\ accidental\ pregnancies}{Total\ months\ of\ exposure} \times 1200$$

$$PI = \frac{20}{2400} \times 1200 = 10\ per\ HWY.$$

4. **In a village with 180 eligible couples, family planning data of contraceptive methods is:** Vasectomy—3, tubectomy—8, IUD users—10, Oral pills—10, condom users—29. Calculate the effective couple protection rate in the village.
   {Hint: Effective protection rates of—sterilization = 100%, IUD= 95%, pills = 100%, condom = 50%}

Ans.

$$Couple\ protection\ rate = \frac{3 + 8 + 10 + 10 + 29}{180} = 33.3\%$$

Taking into account, the effectiveness of contraceptive methods,

Vasectomy—3 (100% of 3), tubectomy—8 (100% of 8), IUD users—9.5 (95% of 10), oral pills—10 (10% of 10), condom users—14.5 (50% of 29)

$$Effective\ couple\ protection\ rate = \frac{3 + 8 + 9.5 + 10 + 14.5}{180} = 25\%$$

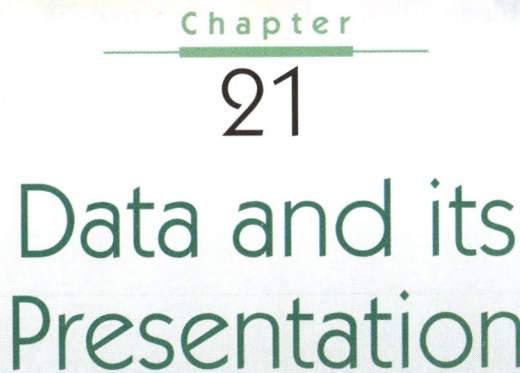

Chapter

21

Data and its Presentation

Competency		Suggested teaching	Suggested assessment
CM6.2	Describe and discuss the principles and demonstrate the methods of collection, classification, analysis, interpretation and presentation of statistical data	Lecture, small group discussion, DOAP sessions	Written/viva voce/skill assessment
CM6.3	Describe, discuss and demonstrate the application of elementary statistical methods including test of significance in various study designs	Lecture, small group discussion, DOAP sessions	Written/viva voce/skill assessment
CM7.4	Define, calculate and interpret morbidity and mortality indicators based on given set of data	Small group, DOAP sessions	Written/skill assessment

1. **Draw the appropriate chart for presenting the causes of worldwide deaths in following table:**

S.No.	Disease	Proportion (%)
1.	CVD	48
2.	Infectious diseases	26
3.	Cancer	22
4.	Accident	04

Ans. Pie chart

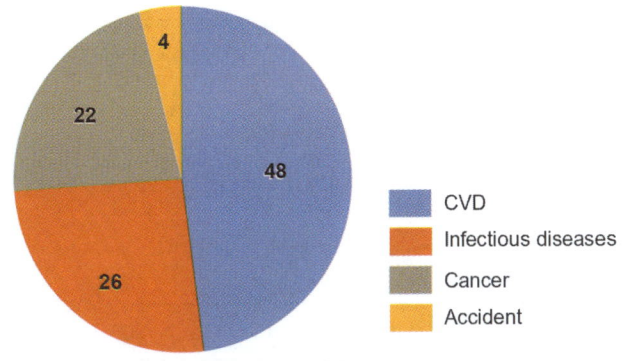

2. **Draw the appropriate chart for decade-wise birth and death rates in India.**

Decade	1901–11	11–21	21–31	31–41	41–51	51–61	61–71	71–81	81–91	91–01
Birth rate	49.2	48.1	46.4	45.2	39.9	41.7	41.2	37.2	32.5	25.0
Death rate	42.6	47.2	36.3	31.2	27.4	22.8	19.0	15.0	11.4	8.1

Ans. Multiple bar chart

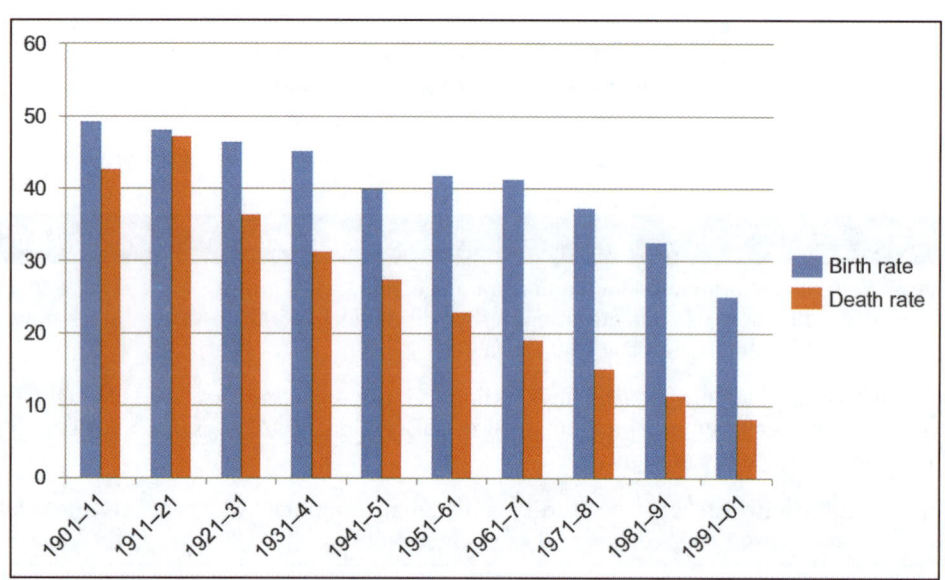

3. **Draw the appropriate chart for showing the correlation between systolic BP and salt intake from following data:**

Salt intake	3.5	5.2	6.9	7.2	8.8
Systolic BP	120	130	140	150	160

Ans. Scatter diagram

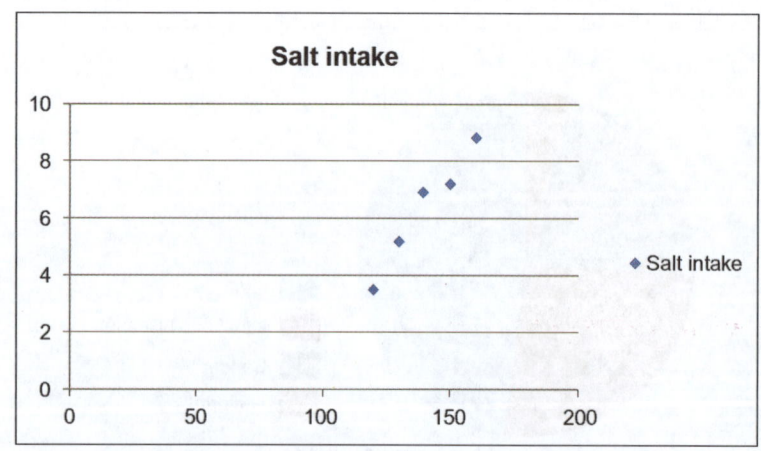

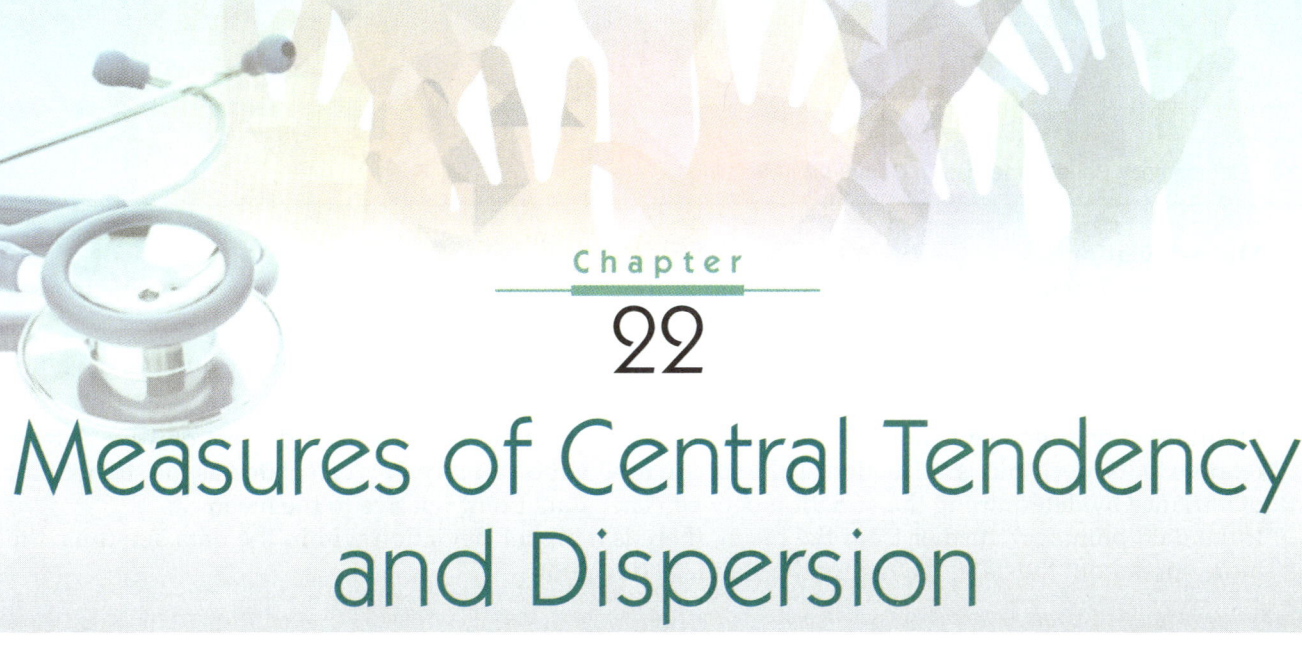

22

Measures of Central Tendency and Dispersion

Competency		Suggested teaching	Suggested assessment
CM6.4	Enumerate, discuss and demonstrate common sampling techniques, simple statistical methods, frequency distribution, measures of central tendency and dispersion	Lecture, small group discussion, DOAP sessions	Written/viva voce/ Skill assessment

Measures of Central Tendency

1. **Mean:** Observations are added and then divided by the number of observations.

2. **Median:** The data is first arranged in an ascending or descending order of magnitude and then the value of middle observation is located.

3. **Mode:** The mode is the commonly occurring value in the distribution of data.

1. **Calculate the mean, median, mode, and range for the following list of values: 13, 18, 13, 14, 13, 16, 14, 21, 13**

Ans.

○ **Mean:** The mean is the usual average, so: 13 + 18 + 13 + 14 + 13 + 16 + 14 + 21 + 13/9 = 15

○ **Median:** The median is the middle value: 13, 13, 13, 13, 14, 14, 16, 18, 21 = The median is 14 (5th number)

○ **Mode:** The mode is the number that is repeated most frequently, so 13 is the mode.

○ **Range:** The largest value in the list is 21, and the smallest is 13, so the range is 21 − 13 = 8.

Measures of Dispersion

1. **Range:** The difference between the highest and lowest figures in a given sample

$$MD = \frac{1}{n}\sum_{i=0}^{n}\left|x_i - \bar{x}\right|$$

2. **Mean deviation:**
   - Absolute differences (differences expressed without plus or minus sign) between each value in a set of values, and the average of all values of that set.
   - Also called mean absolute deviation, it is used as a measure of dispersion where the number of values or quantities is small, otherwise standard deviation is used.

3. **Standard deviation:** The standard deviation is a statistic that measures the dispersion of a dataset relative to its mean and is calculated as the square root of the variance. It is calculated as the square root of variance by determining the variation between each data point relative to the mean.
   If the data points are further from the mean, there is a higher deviation within the data set; thus, the more spread out the data, the higher the standard deviation.

$$SD = \sqrt{\frac{\sum |x - \mu|^2}{N}}$$

4. **Standard error:** The standard error is the approximate standard deviation of a statistical sample population. The standard error is a statistical term that measures the accuracy with which a sample represents a population. In statistics, a sample mean deviates from the actual mean of a population; this deviation is the standard error.

$$SE = \frac{\sigma}{\sqrt{n}}$$

5. **Normal distribution:** The normal distribution can be understood with an example:
   If we collect hemoglobin values of a very large number of people and make a frequency distribution with narrow class intervals, we are likely to get a smooth symmetrical curve. This curve is called a normal distribution curve.

The empirical rule tells what percentage of data falls within a certain number of standard deviations from the mean:
   - 68.2% of the data falls within one standard deviation of the mean.
   - 95.4% of the data falls within two standard deviations of the mean.
   - 99.7% of the data falls within three standard deviations of the mean.

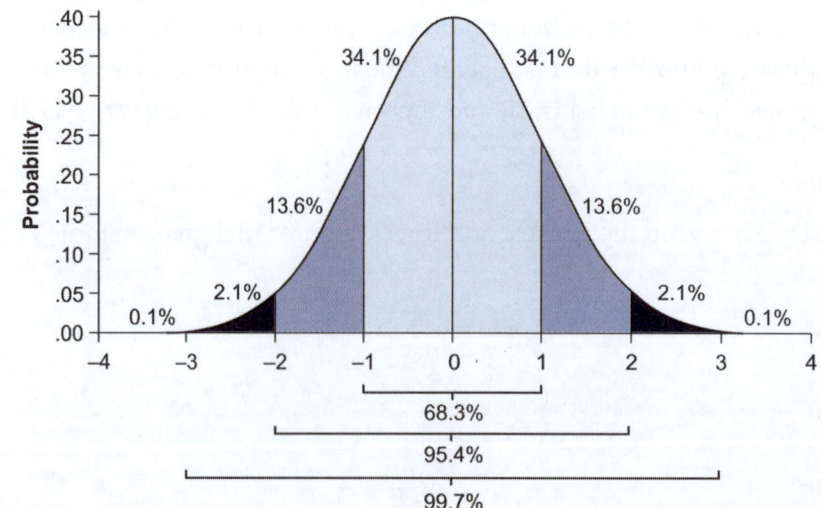

There is a standardized normal curve to estimate the area under curve between any two ordinates. The standard normal curve is a smooth, bell-shaped, symmetrical curve based on an infinitely large number of observations.

The total area of this curve is 1; mean is zero; standard deviation is 1; mean, median, mode coincide

The distance of a value (x) from the mean of the curve (μ) in units of standard deviation is called "relative deviate or standard normal variate" denoted by Z

$$Z = \frac{(x - \mu)}{\text{Standard deviation}}$$

Skewness of Data

Skewness refers to the lack of symmetry. A distribution, or data set, is symmetric if it looks the same to the left and right of the centre point. The skewness for a normal distribution is zero. However, asymmetric data can be left skewed or right skewed.

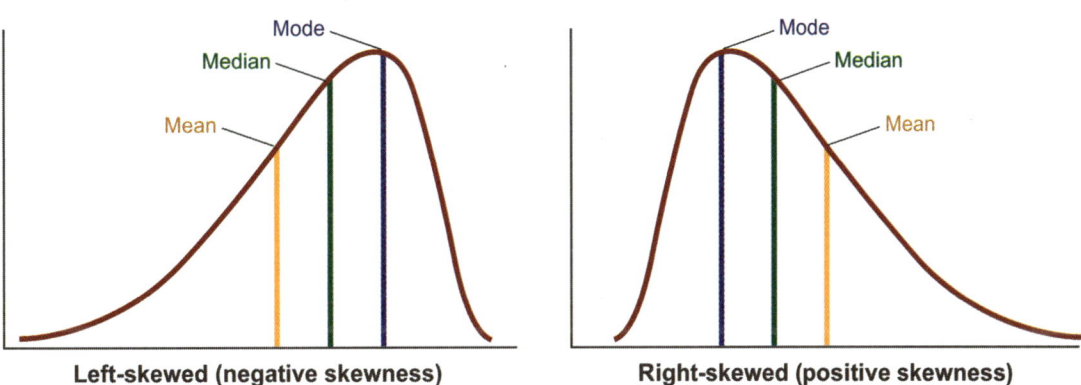

| Left-skewed (negative skewness) | Right-skewed (positive skewness) |

2. **Calculate the standard deviation (SD) of the following data series 4, 9, 11, 12, 17, 5, 8, 12, 14**

Ans.

- First, calculate the mean: 10.2
- Now, subtract the mean individually from each of the numbers given and square the result.
- Now add up these results: 139.55
- Divide it by the number of values, so in this case is 9. This gives us: 15.51
- And finally, square root this to get SD: 3.94

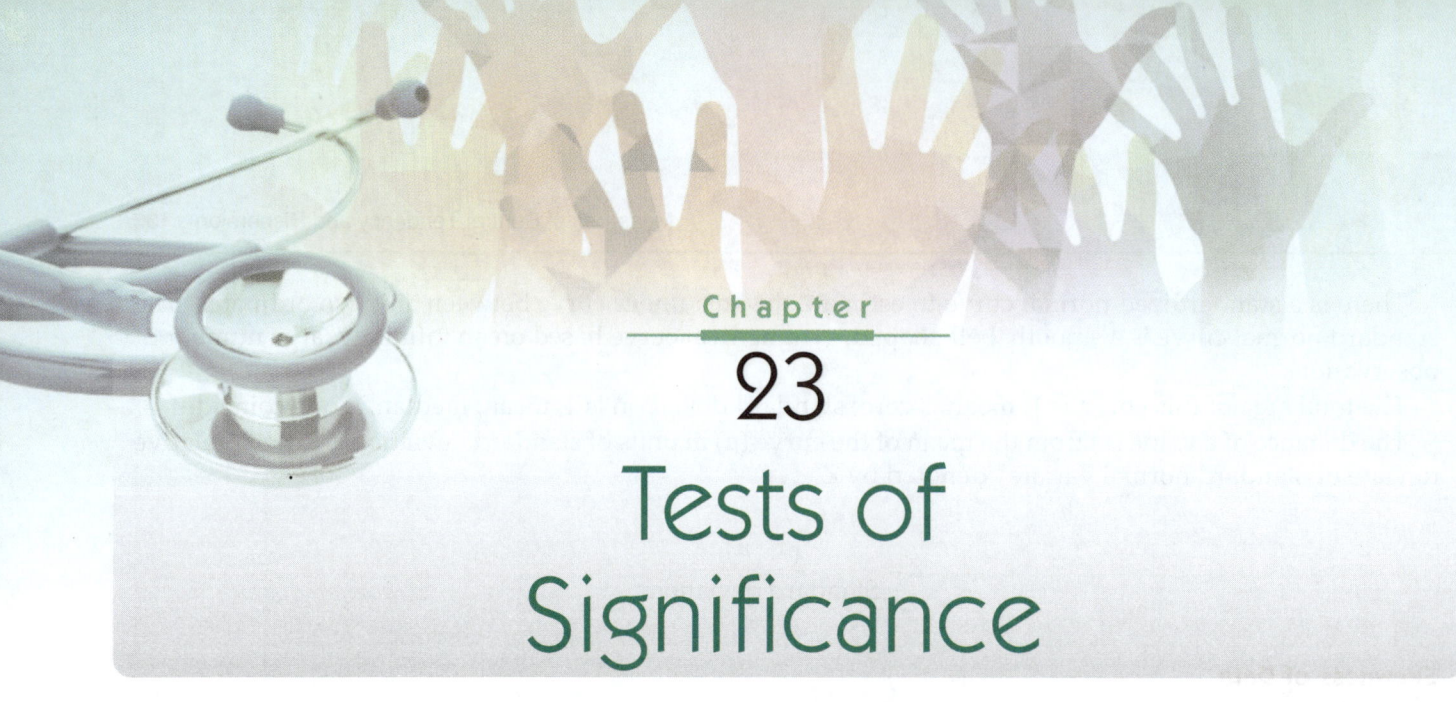

23

Tests of Significance

Competency		Suggested teaching	Suggested assessment
CM6.4	Enumerate, discuss and demonstrate common sampling techniques, simple statistical methods, frequency distribution, measures of central tendency and dispersion	Lecture, small group discussion, DOAP sessions	Written/viva voce/skill assessment

A test of significance is a formal procedure for comparing observed data with a claim (also called a hypothesis), the truth of which is being assessed.

○ The claim is a statement about a parameter, like the population proportion p or the population mean μ.

○ The results of a significance test are expressed in terms of a probability that measures how well the data and the claim agree.

Tests of statistical significance can be divided broadly into four categories:

1. Standard error of the mean

2. Standard error of proportion

3. Standard error of difference

4. Standard error of difference between proportions

Steps in Significance Testing (4-Step Process)

1. State the null and alternative hypotheses.

2. Calculate the test statistic.

3. Find the P-value (using a table or statistical software).

4. Compare P-value with α and decide whether the null hypothesis should be rejected or accepted.

Null Hypothesis

It can be understood with the following example:

- **The null hypothesis:** H_0: Application of bio-fertilizer does not increase plant growth
- **Alternate hypothesis:** H_A: Application of bio-fertilizer increase plant growth

Researchers work to reject, nullify or disprove the null hypothesis. Researchers come up with an alternate hypothesis, one that they think explains a phenomenon, and then work to reject the null hypothesis.

- **Type I error:** It is rejecting the null hypothesis which is true. Also known as α error showing false positive results.
- **Type II error:** It is not rejecting the null hypothesis which is false. Also known as β error showing false negative results.
- **1–β error:** Power of the test to detect a disease, e.g. $\beta = 20$, power $(1-\beta) = 80\%$, probability of correctly detecting the difference between the treatments if the treatments do in fact differ
- **P value,** P= 0.05 means that there is a 5% chance that our observation is false.

Chi-Square Test

It offers an alternate method of testing the significance of difference between two proportions.

Steps

1. Test the null hypothesis
2. Apply chi-square test
3. Finding degree of freedom: df = (c–1) (r–1); c= no. of columns; r= no. of rows
4. Probability tables

Table 22.1: Critical values of the Chi-square distribution with d degrees of freedom

	Probability of exceeding the critical value						
d	0.05	0.01	0.001	d	0.05	0.01	0.001
1	3.841	6.635	10.828	11	19.675	24.725	31.264
2	5.991	9.210	13.816	12	21.026	26.217	32.910
3	7.815	11.345	16.266	13	22.362	27.688	34.528
4	9.488	13.277	18.467	14	23.685	29.141	36.123
5	11.070	15.086	20.515	15	24.996	30.578	37.697
6	12.592	16.812	22.458	16	26.296	32.000	39.252
7	14.067	18.475	24.322	17	27.587	33.409	40.790
8	15.507	20.090	26.125	18	28.869	34.805	42.312
9	16.919	21.666	27.877	19	30.144	36.191	43.820
10	18.307	23.209	29.588	20	31.410	37.566	45.315

1. **A study was conducted in a hospital. The researcher asked about the history of usage of iron supplements from the mothers with low birth weight babies and compared with normal births.**

Iron supplements use	Birth weight		Total
	< 2500 g	> 2500 g	
Yes	40 (a)	80 (b)	120
No	60 (c)	20 (d)	80
Total	100	100	200

   a. *Name of the study design*

Ans. Case control study

   b. *What type of statistical test will you use to find any association between maternal intake of iron supplements and low birth weight?*

Ans. Chi-square test will be used to find the association

H_0 = No association between iron intake and birth weight

H_1 = There is association between the two.

Level of significance 5%

   c. *Is there any statistically significant association between maternal intake of iron supplements and low birth weight?*

Ans. $\chi^2 = \dfrac{(O-E)^2}{E}$

O = Observed value, E = Expected value

χ^2 value for each cell has to be calculated.

$$E \text{ for each cell} = \frac{\text{Column or vertical total} \times \text{Row or horizontal total}}{\text{Sample total}}$$

For example, E for a cell = $\dfrac{100 \times 120}{200}$ = 60

χ^2 for 'a' = $\dfrac{(40-60)^2}{60}$ = 6.67

Total χ^2 = χ^2 for 'a' + χ^2 for 'b' + χ^2 for 'c' + χ^2 for 'd'

Also, $\chi^2 = \dfrac{(ad-bc)^2(a+b+c+d)}{(a+b)(c+d)(a+c)(b+d)}$

$\chi^2 = \dfrac{(40 \times 20 - 80 \times 60)^2(40+80+60+20)}{(40+80)(60+20)(40+60)(80+20)}$

χ^2 = 33.33

Degree of freedom = (r–1) (c–1) = (2–1) (2–1) = 1

At one degree of freedom, χ^2 value corresponding to probability 0.05 is 3.841. Calculated value 33.33 is higher, hence significant at 5% level. Thus there is significant difference between the iron intake and birth weight.

2. **A group of 50 diabetic patients were divided into two equal groups to test the effect of a new antidiabetic drug. Group A was the control group, i.e. old drug. The other group, B was given new drug. At the end of 2 months, fasting blood sugar levels were tested and following observations were made:**

	Number	Mean	Standard deviation
Group A	25	170	10.1
Group B	25	124	22.4

a. *Can you conclude that the new drug significantly decreased sugar levels as compared to old drug? What type of test will you use here?*

Ans. A screening test was done for cervical cancer. Results are given below.

b. *Can you conclude that the new drug significantly decreased sugar levels as compared to old drug? What type of test will you use here?*

Ans. t test or standard error (SE) of difference between two means will be used here

SE = $\sqrt{(\alpha_1)^2/n_1 + (\alpha_2)^2/n_2}$

= $\sqrt{(10.1)^2/25 + (22.4)^2/25}$

= $\sqrt{24.9}$

= 4.98

The standard error of difference between the two means is (170–124) = 46, which is more than twice the standard error of difference between the two means, and therefore "significant." It can be concluded that the new drug significantly decreases blood sugar levels as compared to old drug.

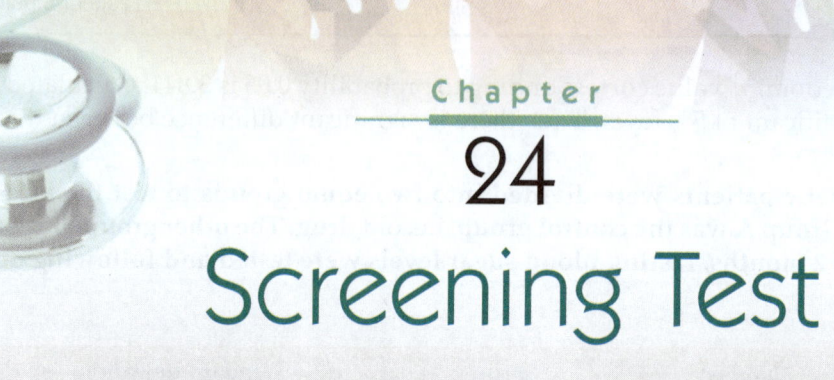

Chapter

24

Screening Test

Competency		Suggested teaching	Suggested assessment
CM7.6	Enumerate and evaluate the need of screening tests	Lecture, small group discussion, DOAP sessions	Written/viva voce/skill assessment

Screening

Screening is defined as the presumptive identification of unrecognized disease in an apparently healthy, asymptomatic population by means of tests, examinations or other procedures that can be applied rapidly and easily to the target population. e.g.: Pap smear testing for cervical cancer, Hb testing during ANC for anemia.

Characteristics of a screening test:
1. Important health problem.
2. Treatment available.
3. Confirmatory test available.
4. Asymptomatic or latent stage in disease.
5. Acceptable.
6. Natural history of disease adequately understood.
7. Agreed policy on treatment.
8. Affordable.
9. Sensitive.
10. Ease of application.

1. **Calculate the sensitivity, specificity of the test. Find the false positive, false negative rate. Also calculate predictive value of positive and negative test.**

Screening test PAP smear	Disease positive	Disease negative	Total
Test positive	400(a)	150(b)	550
Test negative	100(c)	4350(d)	4450
Total	500	4500	5000

Sensitivity = a/a+c =400/500 = 80%

     = a (true positive)/a+c (true positive + false negative)

     = Probability of being test positive when disease present

Specificity = d/b+d = 4350/4500 = 96%

     = d (true negative)/b+d (true negative + false positive)

     = Probability of being test negative when disease absent

  PPV: = a/a+b = 400/550 = 73%

     = a (true positive)/a+b (true positive + false positive)

     = Probability (patient having disease when test is positive)

  NPV: = d/c+d = 98%

     = d (true negative)/c+d (false negative + true negative)

     = Probability (patient not having disease when test is negative)

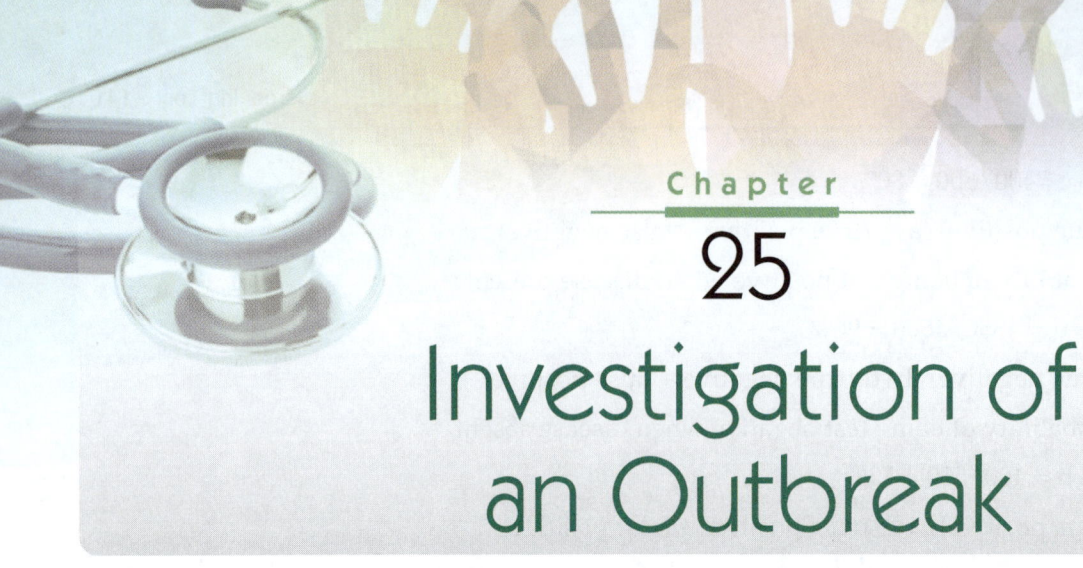

Investigation of
an Outbreak

Competency	Suggested teaching	Suggested assessment
CM20.2 Describe various issues during outbreaks and their prevention	Lecture, small group discussion	Written/viva voce

Investigating An Outbreak/Epidemic

It is a set of procedures used to identify the cause responsible for the disease, the people affected, the circumstances and mode of spread of the disease, and other relevant factors involved in propagating the epidemic, and to take effective actions to contain and prevent the spread of the disease.

Objectives of Outbreak Investigation

1. Control or prevention of the health problem.

2. Opportunity to learn (research opportunity).

3. Public, political, or legal concerns

4. Public health program considerations

5. Training

    1. **A total number of 84 out of 500 hosteller students developed diphtheria illness and 2 died due to it. The day wise distribution of occurrence of diphtheria is as follows:**

    Day 1 = 1 case

    Day 6 = 9 cases

    Day 7 = 12 cases

    a. *How many cases are primary and secondary?*

Ans. Primary (1), Secondary (21)

b. *Calculate the attack rate.*

$$\text{Attack rate} = \frac{\text{Number of new cases of a specified disease during a specified time interval}}{\text{Total population at risk during the same time interval}} \times 100$$

AR = 84/500 *100 = 16.8

c. *Calculate the secondary attack rate.*

$$\text{SAR} = \frac{\text{Number of exposed persons developing the disease within the range of incubation period}}{\text{Total number of exposed/ susceptible contacts}} \times 100$$

SAR = 21/499 * 100 = 4.2

d. *Calculate the case fatality rate.*

$$\text{Case fatality rate} = \frac{\text{Total no. of deaths due to a particular disease}}{\text{Total no. of cases due to the same disease}} \times 100$$

CFR = 2/84 *100 = 2.3

e. *Define an epidemic. Write the steps of outbreak investigation.*

Epidemic: The occurrence in a community or region of cases of an illness, specific health-related behavior, or health-related events clearly in excess of normal expectancy.

Steps:

1. Verification of diagnosis
2. Confirmation of the existence of an epidemic
3. Defining the population at risk
4. Rapid search for all cases and their characteristics
5. Data analysis
6. Formulation of hypotheses
7. Testing of hypotheses
8. Evaluation of ecological factors
9. Further investigation of population at risk
10. Writing the report.

BIBLIOGRAPHY

1. Charley Kyd, MBA Microsoft Excel MVP, 2005–2014
2. Dept. of Community Medicine, Geetanjali Medical College and Hospital, Udaipur.
3. https://www.statisticshowto.datasciencecentral.com/pearson-mode-skewness/
4. Introduction to population genetics, D.1, 2013 Sinauer Associates. Inc
5. Park K. Environmental and Health. In Park's Textbook of Preventive and Social Medicine, 25th ed. Jabalpur, India: M/S Banarsidas Bhanot Publishers; 2019.

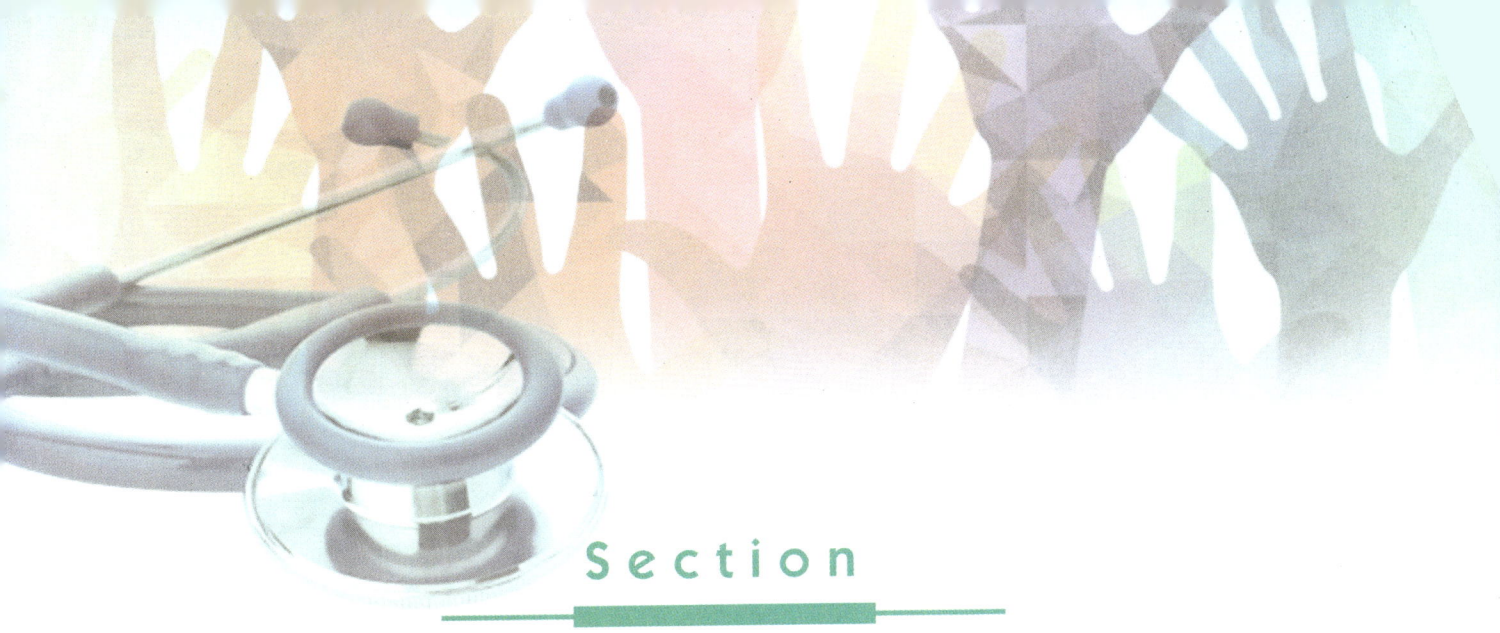

Section

IV
Field Visits to Public Health Institutions

- ◈ Milk Processing Unit (Dairy)
- ◈ District Health Store (Cold Chain)
- ◈ District Tuberculosis Centre
- ◈ Biomedical Waste Management Facility
- ◈ Anganwadi Centre (ICDS Scheme)
- ◈ Non-governmental Health Agency (NGO)
- ◈ Immunization Clinic
- ◈ Subcentre
- ◈ Primary Health Centre
- ◈ Community Health Centre
- ◈ Urban Health Training Centre (UHTC)
- ◈ Rural Health Training Centre (RHTC)
- ◈ Industrial Unit

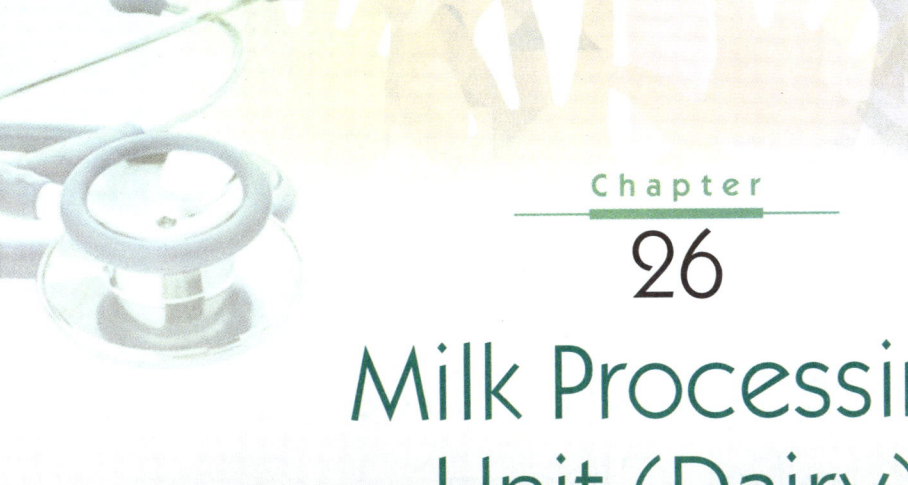

26

Milk Processing Unit (Dairy)

Competency		Suggested teaching	Suggested assessment
CM5.7	Describe food hygiene (milk)	Lecture, small group discussion	Written/viva voce

Brief Description of the Unit

Milk is initially collected from milk vans and checked for purity and quality. It is then transported to the plants where it is transferred to huge tanks. The milk is then separated and clarified. After the clarification process, it is then processed again to separate full cream milk and toned milk. The process of segregation is followed by the addition of fortified minerals and vitamins in the milk. The product is then made ready for pasteurization. The pasteurized milk is then homogenized to remove the fat content from the milk. It is then packaged and sold to the consumer markets.

How is Milk Pasteurized?

Pasteurization involves rapidly heating milk (to less than the boiling point), maintaining it uniformly over a definite period and rapidly cooling it. This destroys most of the pathogenic microorganisms, reduces the total quantity of all the microorganisms without affecting its inherent qualities (taste and flavour).

The methods of pasteurizing milk are as follows:

    a. *Holder (Vat) method:* Temperatures between 63°C and 65.5° C and holding it for 30 min before cooling it rapidly to 5 C.

    b. *High temperature short time (HTST) method:* Temperature of 72 C for 15 seconds and then rapidly cooled to 4°C.

    c. *Ultra high temperature (UHT) method:* Temperature under pressure, between 125°C and 150° C for a few seconds only and then rapidly cooled.

How will you Check for the Efficiency of Pasteurization?

Phosphatase test: This test is meant for ascertaining the efficiency of pasteurization and depends on the fact that the enzyme phosphatase is destroyed by the pasteurization temperatures.

147

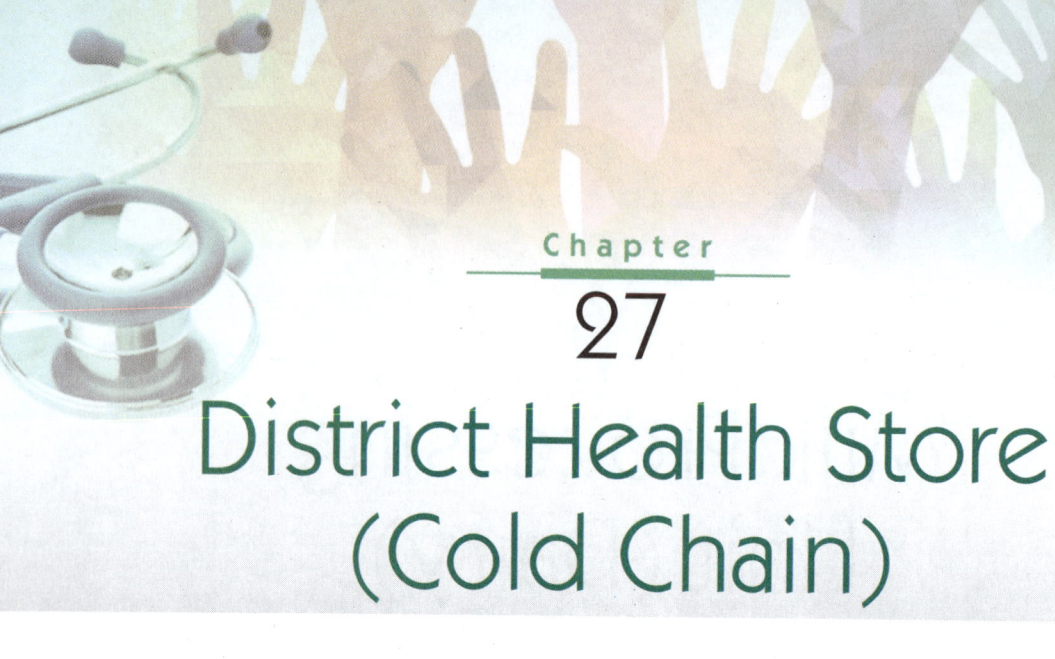

27

District Health Store (Cold Chain)

Competency		Suggested teaching	Suggested assessment
PE19.3	Vaccine description with regard to classification of vaccines, strain used, dose, route, schedule, risks, benefits and side effects, indications and contraindications	Lecture, small group discussion	Written/viva voce
PE19.4	Define cold chain and discuss the methods of safe storage and handling of vaccines	Lecture, small group discussion	Written/viva voce

Brief Description of the Store

District medical store is responsible for procurement and storage of medical stores for dependent hospitals. The depots receive stores from various suppliers and make local purchase of stores. There are norms for provisioning and procurement of medical items by the depots to avoid overstocking. For storage of medical stores, three types of facilities are required, viz. cold room, cool room, and day temperature room facility.

Write down about Cold Chain Equipment present at the Store

1. Cold and freezer rooms and/or freezers,
2. Ice lined refrigerators
3. Deep freezers
4. Cold boxes
5. Temperature monitoring equipment.

What is Reverse Cold Chain?

Reverse cold chain is the process of maintaining the cold chain when heat sensitive items are stored and transported in the reverse direction, i.e. upwards from the clinic to a depot or laboratory. This process is also used for transporting specimen samples. It is used in acute flaccid paralysis (AFP) surveillance in polio eradication program to carry out the stool sample of suspected case.

How are Various Vaccines Stored at the store?

1. At the health centre, most vaccines (except polio) can be stored up to 5 weeks if the refrigerator temperature is strictly kept at +2°C to +8°C.
2. Cold compartment: "T" series (DPT, TT, DT), hepatitis B, Hib vaccine, BCG and diluents.
3. Freezer compartment: Polio and Measles (P and M)
4. Reconstituted BCG vaccine and measles vaccine can be kept at +2°C to +8°C for maximum 4 hours and JE vaccine for 2 hours.

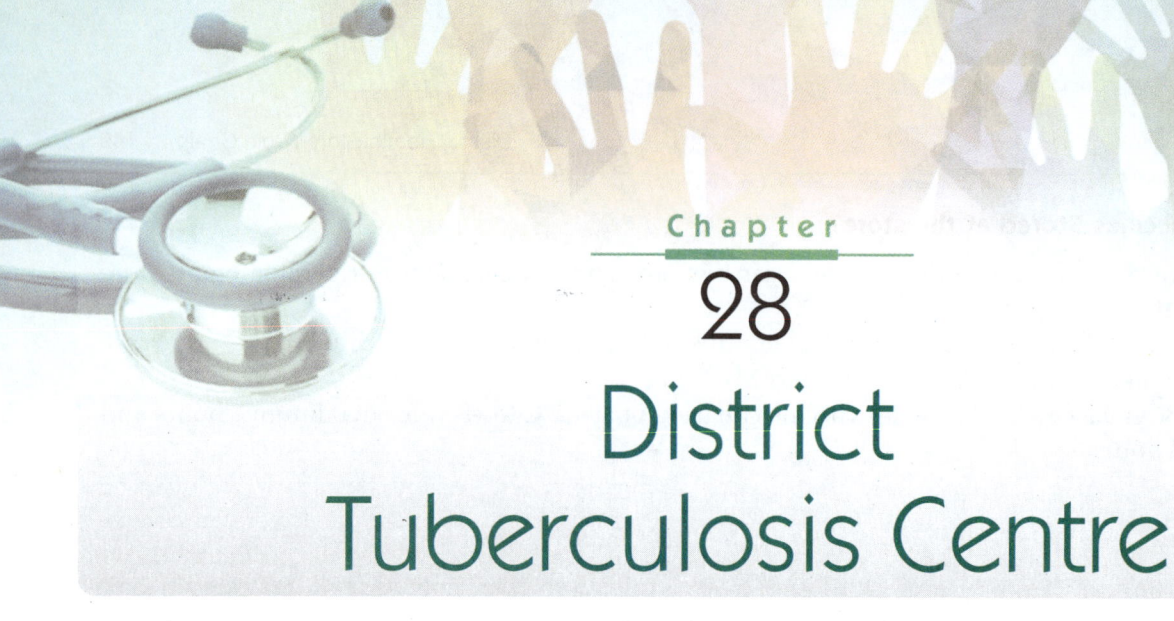

28

District
Tuberculosis Centre

Competency		Suggested teaching	Suggested assessment
PH1.55	Describe and discuss the following National Health Programmes including tuberculosis.	Lecture, small group discussion	Written/viva voce
PE34.3	Discuss the various regimens for management of tuberculosis as per National Guidelines	Lecture, small group discussion	Written/viva voce
PE34.4	Discuss the preventive strategies adopted and the objectives and outcome of the National Tuberculosis Control Program	Lecture, small group discussion	Written/viva voce
CT1.1	Describe and discuss the epidemiology of tuberculosis and its impact on the work, life and economy of India	Lecture, small group discussion	Written/viva voce
CT1.4	Describe the epidemiology, the predisposing factors and microbial and therapeutic factors that determine resistance to drugs	Lecture, small group discussion	Written/viva voce
CT1.15	Prescribe an appropriate antituberculosis regimen based on the location of disease, smear positivity and negativity and comorbidities based on current national guidelines including directly observed tuberculosis therapy (DOTS)	Bedside clinic, small group discussion, lecture	Skill assessment
CT1.18	Educate health care workers on national programs of tuberculosis and administering and monitoring the DOTS program	DOAP (Demonstration, Observation, Assistance and Performance) session	Skill assessment

Brief Description of the Centre

District TB centre has 20 to 100 TB beds usually under the charge of a medical officer/district TB Officer or TB/chest physician. District TB centre have facilities for direct microscopy; many are also equipped with X-ray/CBNAAT with necessary technicians for diagnostic activity. A TB health visitor or two may also be there, in addition to the (drug) dispenser and other ancillary staff.

Write down about the Treatment Boxes Present at the Centre

The TB drugs for RNTCP patients are supplied in an individual patient wise box which contains the entire course of treatment for the patient. In each patient wise box there are two pouches. One is for the intensive phase and the other is for the continuation phase. The patient wise boxes are color coded. Previously red boxes were for new patients, and blue boxes are for previously treated patients. For pediatric TB patients separate patient wise boxes have been developed.

What are the Recent Techniques of Diagnosing TB?

1. Interferon Gamma Release Assay (IGRA)
2. Fluorescent microscopy
3. GeneXpert test and the TrueNat test (CBNAAT)

What is MDR TB?

A TB patient whose biological specimen is resistant to both INH and rifampicin with or without resistance other first-line ATD, based on results from a quality assured laboratory.

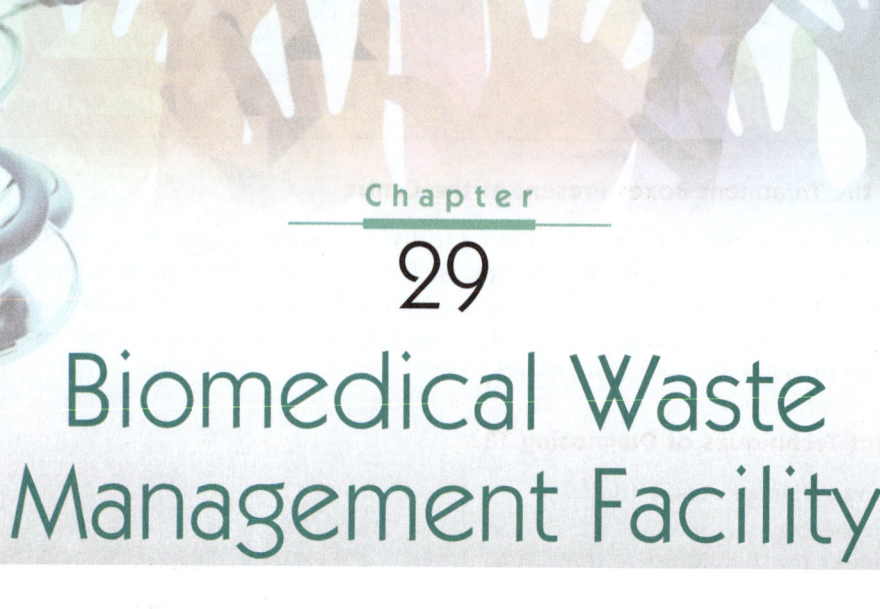

Chapter

29

Biomedical Waste Management Facility

Competency		Suggested teaching	Suggested assessment
CM14.1	Define and classify hospital waste	Lecture, small group discussion, visit to hospital	Written/viva voce
CM14.2	Describe various methods of treatment of hospital waste	Lecture, small group discussion, visit to hospital	Written/viva voce
CM14.3	Describe laws related to hospital waste management	Lecture, small group discussion	Written/viva voce

What is Biomedical Waste?

"Bio-medical waste" means any waste, which is generated during the diagnosis, treatment or immunization of human beings or animals or research activities pertaining thereto or in the production or testing of biological or in health camps.

What are the Various Types of Waste Categories and Disposal Bags?

Category	Type of waste	
Yellow	✗ Human anatomical waste ✗ Animal anatomical waste ✗ Soiled waste ✗ Discarded linen, mattresses, beddings contaminated with blood or body fluid.	✗ Discarded of expired medicine ✗ Chemical waste ✗ Chemical liquid waste ✗ Microbiology, biotechnology and other clinical laboratory waste (pre-treated)
Red	✗ Contaminated waste (Recyclable)	
White	✗ Waste sharps including metals	
Blue	✗ Glassware	
	✗ Metallic body implants	

Ref: Ministry of Environment, Forest and Climate Change, (2018) Biomedical waste management rules.

What is Composition of Biomedical Waste Committee?

It includes:
- SMO/CMO/Medical Superintendent (Chairperson)
- District Quality Consultant/District BMW Officer (Invitee Members)
- Quality Manager
- Hospital Infection Control Nurse/Officer
- Nursing Incharge
- Medical Officer (Surgery)
- Medical Officer (Emergency)
- Medical Officer (Gynae and Obs)
- Microbiologist/Pathologist
- OT Nurse/Technician/Assistant
- Lab Technician
- Blood Bank/Storage Unit Technician
- Housekeeping Incharge
- Pharmacist

What are Various Techniques of Biomedical Waste Disposal?

Chemical disinfection, incineration, autoclaving, microwaving, shredding, pulverization and secured landfill.

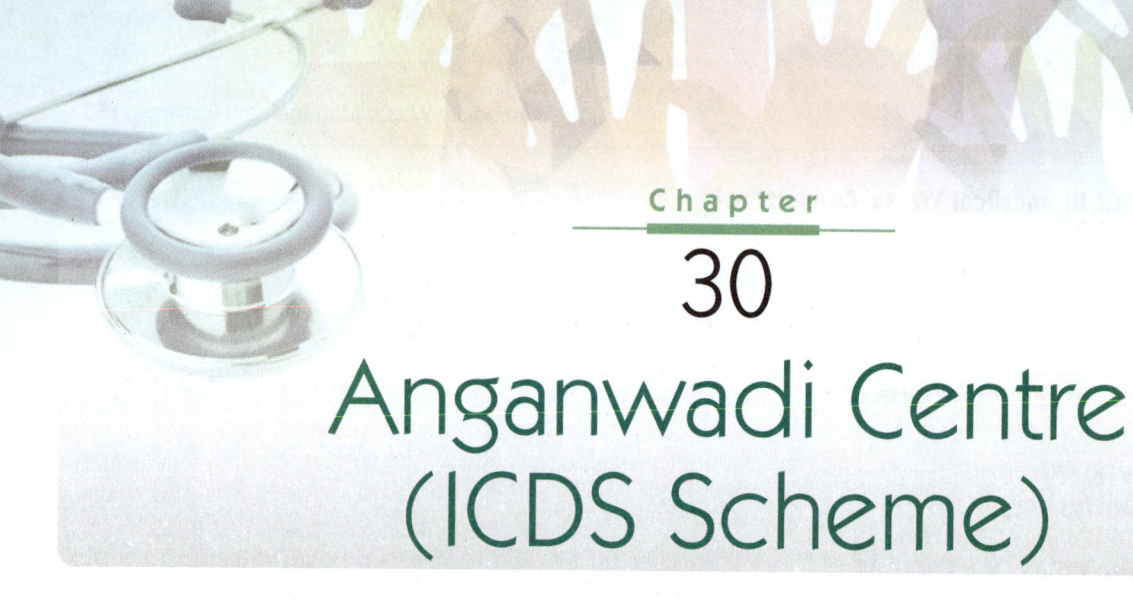

Anganwadi Centre (ICDS Scheme)

Competency		Suggested teaching	Suggested assessment
CM5.6	Enumerate and discuss the National Nutrition Policy, important national nutritional programs including the Integrated Child Development Services (ICDS) Scheme, etc	Lecture, small group discussion	Written/viva voce
CM5.2	Describe and demonstrate the correct method of performing a nutritional assessment of individuals, families and the community by using the appropriate method	DOAP	OSCE

Services Provided at the Centre

1. Supplementary nutrition
2. Non-formal pre-school education
3. Immunization
4. Health check-up
5. Referral services
6. Nutrition and health education

Coverage and Staffing at the Centre

150–1000, Anganwadi worker and anganwadi helper.

Beneficiaries at the Centre

1. Children below 6 years
2. Pregnant mothers
3. Lactating mothers
4. Women (15–45 years)
5. Adolescent girls

How is Growth Monitoring of Children Done?

Growth monitoring and nutrition surveillance are two important activities that are undertaken. Children below the age of three years are weighed once a month and children 3–6 years of age are weighed every quarter. Weight-for-age growth cards are maintained for all children below six years. This helps to detect growth faltering and helps in assessing nutritional status.

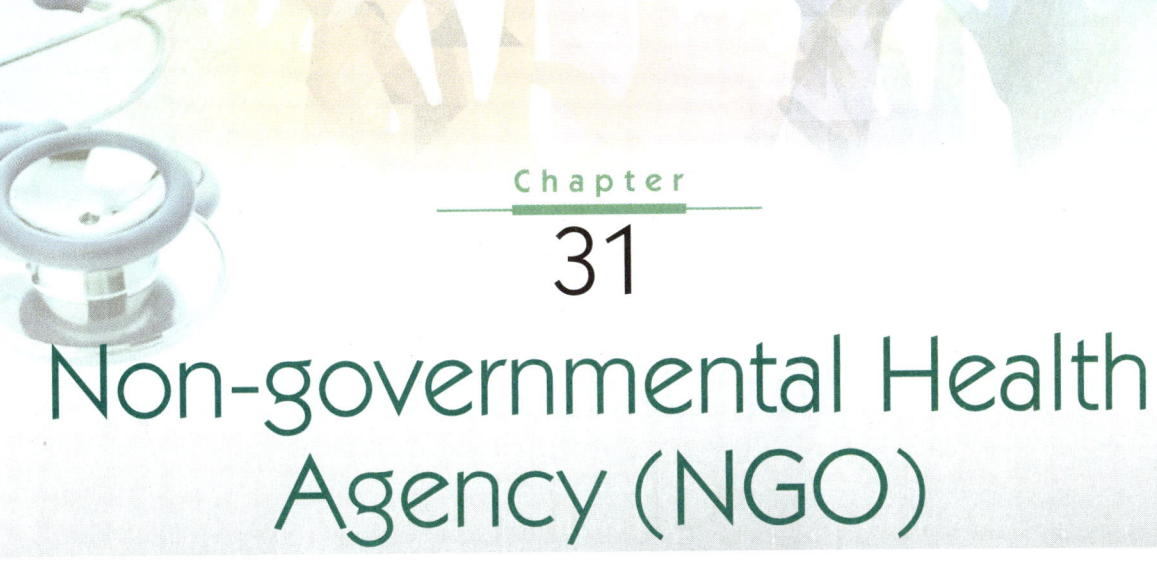

Non-governmental Health Agency (NGO)

Competency		Suggested teaching	Suggested assessment
CM18.1	Define and describe the concept of international health	Lecture, small group discussion	Written/viva voce
CM18.2	Describe roles of various international health agencies	Lecture, small group discussion	Written/viva voce

Description of the NGO

NGOs play a key role in supporting the public health system at grassroot level by enhancing the management of primary health centres and related bodies. Development of effective and efficient models of healthcare service delivery, and NGOs with their willingness to learn and adapt to new challenges can surely take a lead in this direction.

What are the Functions of the NGO?

a. Development of primary health care programs.
b. Comprehensive human development
c. Conduct reviews and assessment of existing health and development programs.
d. Promote full participation by individuals and communities in health planning.
e. Training of health workers, supervisors, administrators, planners, etc.
f. Develop locally sustainable and appropriate health technologies, etc.

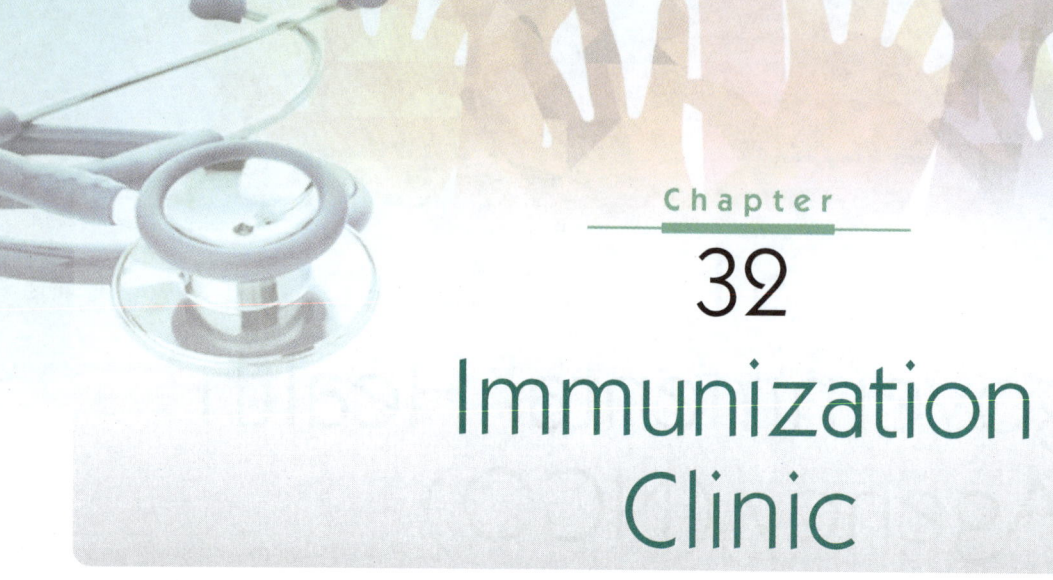

Immunization Clinic

Competency		Suggested teaching	Suggested assessment
PE19.3	Vaccine description with regard to classification of vaccines, strain used, dose, route, schedule, risks, benefits and side effects, indications and contraindications	Lecture, small group discussion	Written/viva voce
PE19.4	Define cold chain and discuss the methods of safe storage and handling of vaccines	Lecture, small group discussion	Written/viva voce
PE19.12	Observe the administration the UIP vaccines	DOAP (Demonstration, Observation, Assistance and Performance) session	Document in log book

Description of the Immunization Clinic

Immunization clinics have proper vaccine storage and handling, dedicated personnel (doctors and nurses) for administering the vaccine and process documentation. The cases are recommended vaccines after appropriate history taking, examination and noting other details of associated medical conditions, allergies etc. Vaccines are recommended as per national guidelines.

Various Types of Injection Techniques

1. Intramuscular (IM) injection administers the vaccine into the muscle mass.
2. Subcutaneous (SC) injection administers the vaccine into the subcutaneous layer above the muscle and below the skin.
3. Intradermal (ID) injection administers the vaccine in the topmost layer of the skin.
4. Oral administration
5. Intranasal flu vaccine

Vaccines Under National Immunization Schedule

BCG, polio (oral/injectable), pentavalent, pneumococcal, rotavirus, hepatitis, tetanus, measles and Japanese encephalitis, etc.

Enlist Measures for Universal Precautions

Universal precautions are simple infection control measures that reduce the risk of transmission of blood-borne pathogens through exposure to blood or body fluids among patients and health care workers. Under the "universal precaution" principle, blood and body fluids from all persons should be considered as potentially infectious, regardless of the known or supposed status of the person.

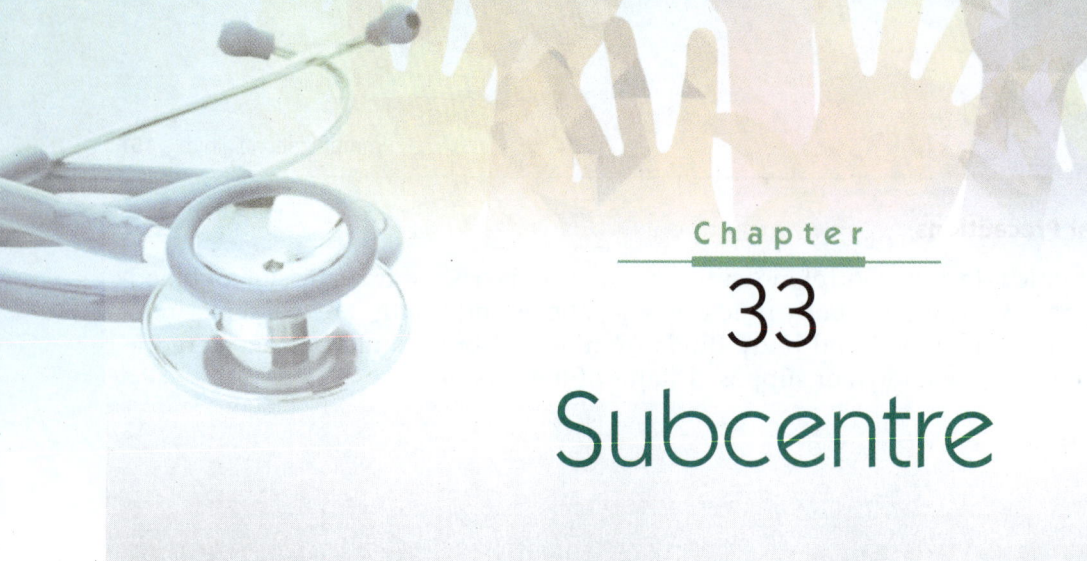

Subcentre

Competency		Suggested teaching	Suggested assessment
CM17.1	Define and describe the concept of health care to community	Lecture, small group discussion	Written/viva voce
CM17.3	Describe primary health care, its components and principles	Lecture, small group discussion	Written/viva voce
CM17.5	Describe health care delivery in India	Lecture, small group discussion	Written/viva voce

Brief Description of the Centre

Subcentre caters to a 3000–5000 population. It is the first contact point between the primary health care system and the community. It covers 3–5 villages each covered by an ASHA worker.

Staff Present at Subcentre

1. Auxiliary nurse midwife (ANM)
2. Male health worker commonly known as multi-purpose worker (male).
3. Voluntary/contract worker.

Services Provided at the Centre

1. Immunization
2. Antenatal, natal and postnatal care
3. Prevention of malnutrition and common childhood diseases
4. Family planning services and counselling.
5. Treatment of minor ailments such as ARI, diarrhea, fever, worm infestation, etc.
6. Community needs assessment.
7. Implementation of national health and family welfare programmes

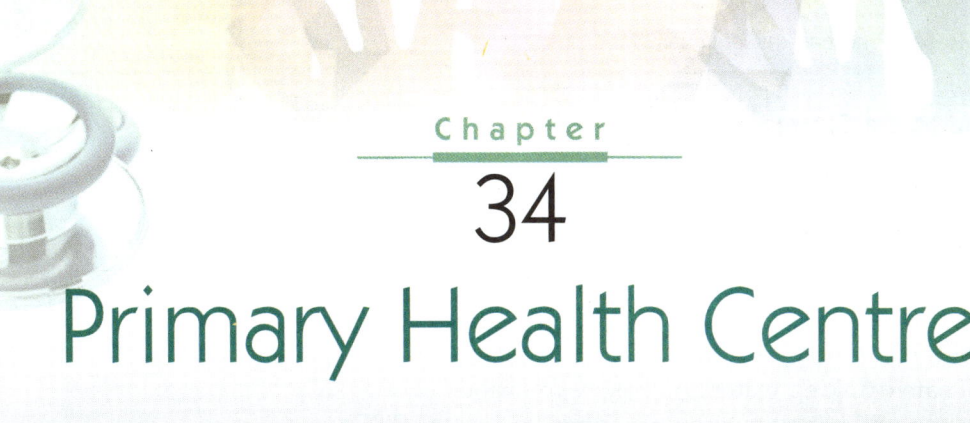

34

Primary Health Centre

Competency		Suggested teaching	Suggested assessment
CM17.1	Define and describe the concept of health care to community	Lecture, small group discussion	Written/viva voce
CM17.3	Describe primary health care, its components and principles	Lecture, small group discussion	Written/viva voce
CM17.5	Describe health care delivery in India	Lecture, small group discussion	Written/viva voce

Brief Description of the Centre

PHC is the first port of call to a qualified doctor of the public sector in rural areas for the sick and those who directly report or referred from subcentres for curative, preventive and promotive health care. It is located in an accessible area well connected for referral and transport.

Staff present at PHC

1. Medical Officer: MBBS
2. MO: AYUSH
3. Accountant/clerk
4. Pharmacist
5. Pharmacist AYUSH
6. Nurse-midwife (staff-nurse)
7. Health workers (F)
8. Health Asstt. (Male)
9. Health Asstt. (Female)/LHV
10. Health educator
11. Data entry-cum-computer operator
12. Laboratory technician
13. Cold chain and vaccine logistic assistant
14. Multi-skilled Group D worker
15. Sanitary worker-cum-watchman

Services Provided at the Centre

1. Medical care
2. MCH care
3. Family welfare
4. Medical termination of pregnancy
5. Nutritional services
6. School health
7. Promotion of safe drinking water and basic sanitation
8. Health education and behaviour change communication (BCC).
9. National programs

Functions of Rogi Kalyan Samiti at PHC

Improvement of the management and service provision of the PHC. It generates its own funds (through users' charges, donation, etc.) and utilize the same for service improvement of the PHC.

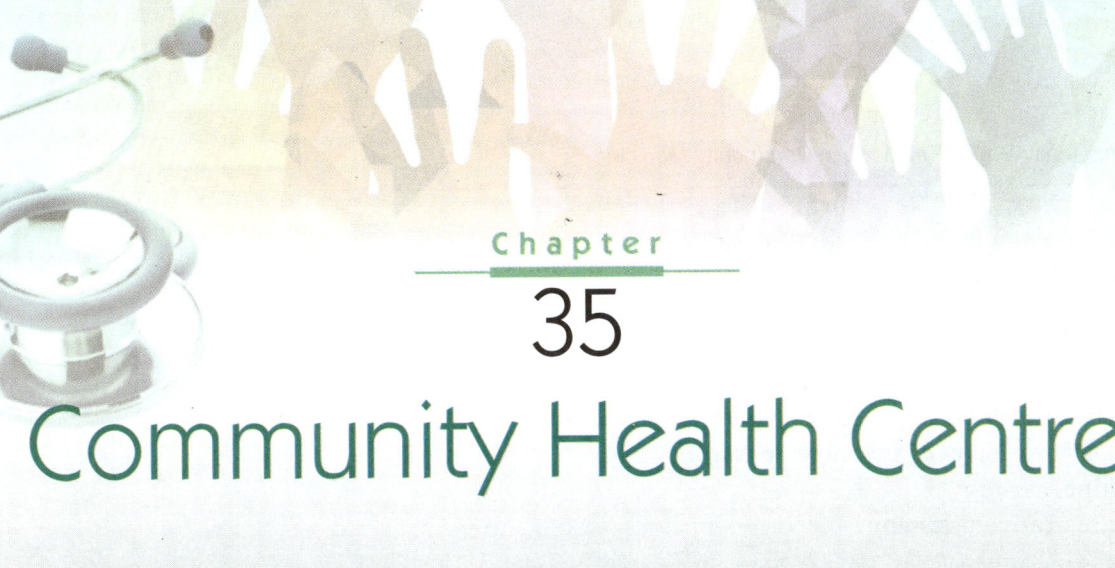

Community Health Centre

Competency		Suggested teaching	Suggested assessment
CM17.1	Define and describe the concept of health care to community	Lecture, small group discussion	Written/viva voce
CM17.3	Describe primary health care, its components and principles	Lecture, small group discussion	Written/viva voce
CM17.5	Describe health care delivery in India	Lecture, small group discussion	Written/viva voce

Brief Description of the Centre

CHC is a block level health administrative unit and gatekeeper for referrals to higher level of facilities. All essential services provided at the CHC are routine and emergency care in surgery, medicine, obstetrics and gynecology, pediatrics, dental and AYUSH in addition to all the National Health Programmes.

Staff Present at CHC

1. Block medical officer/medical superintendent
2. Public health specialist
3. Public health nurse
4. Physician
5. Obstetrician and gynaecologist
6. Pediatrician
7. Anesthetist
8. Medical officer
9. Staff nurse
10. Pharmacist
11. Lab. technician
12. Radiographer
13. Dietician
14. Ophthalmic assistant

15. Dental assistant
16. Cold chain and vaccine logistic assistant
17. OT technician
18. Multi-rehabilitation/community-based rehabilitation worker
19. Counsellor
20. Registration clerk
21. Statistical assistant/data entry operator
22. Account assistant
23. Administrative assistant

Services provided at a CHC

1. OPD-services and IPD services: General, medicine, surgery, cbstetrics and gynecology, pediatrics, dental and AYUSH services.
2. Eye specialist services (at one for every 5 CHCs)
3. Emergency services
4. Laboratory services
5. National Health Programmes

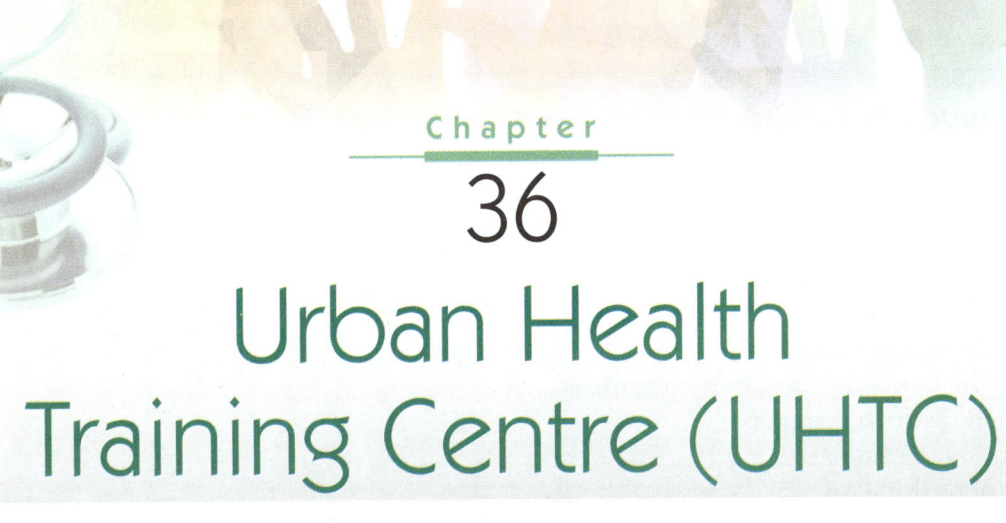

36
Urban Health Training Centre (UHTC)

Competency		Suggested teaching	Suggested assessment
CM17.1	Define and describe the concept of health care to community	Lecture, small group discussion	Written/viva voce
CM17.2	Describe community diagnosis	Lecture, small group discussion	Written/viva voce
CM17.3	Describe primary health care, its components and principles	Lecture, small group discussion	Written/viva voce
CM17.4	Describe national policies related to health and health planning and sustainable development goals	Lecture, small group discussion	Written/viva voce
CM17.5	Describe health care delivery in India	Lecture, small group discussion	Written/viva voce

Brief Description of the Centre

UHTC covers a population of approximately 5000 urban residents. It aims to provide comprehensive health care services to the community along with teaching and training of postgraduate, interns and undergraduate students in urban health.

Staff Present at Centre

1. Medical officer of Health-cum-Lecturer/Assistant Professor
2. Lady medical officer
3. Medical social workers
4. Public health nurse
5. Health inspectors
6. Health educator
7. Technical assistant/technicians
8. Peon
9. Van driver
10. Store keeper
11. Record clerk
12. Sweepers

Functions of UHTC

1. Child health care services: Immunization, nutrition, growth monitoring.
2. Health education of mothers, treatment of minor ailments.
3. Maternal health care services: Antenatal care, nutrition, family planning, education on MCH related matters, contraceptive distribution.
4. Education and training of medical students and interns on primary health care issues.
5. Community health education
6. Participation in national health programmes
7. Survey and research activities.
8. Organization of seminars
9. Training of health workers

Services provided at UHTC

1. Medical care services through outdoor and indoor.
2. Referral services
3. Minor surgery
4. Injection, dressing and drip facility
5. Immunization of child and mother: At AWC, subcentre on MCHN day.
6. ANC check up
7. Family planning and contraceptive distribution
8. Health education
9. Laboratory facility
10. Training and research activities, survey, etc.
11. Specialist services on periodical basis
12. School health programme

Rural Health Training Centre (RHTC)

Competency		Suggested teaching	Suggested assessment
CM17.1	Define and describe the concept of health care to community	Lecture, small group discussion	Written/viva voce
CM17.2	Describe community diagnosis	Lecture, small group discussion	Written/viva voce
CM17.3	Describe primary health care, its components and principles	Lecture, small group discussion	Written/viva voce
CM17.4	Describe national policies related to health and health planning and sustainable development goals	Lecture, small group discussion	Written/viva voce
CM17.5	Describe health care delivery in India	Lecture, small group discussion	Written/viva voce

Brief Description of the Centre

RHTC covers a population of approximately 30,000 rural residents. It aims to provide comprehensive health care services to the community along with teaching and training of postgraduate, interns and undergraduate students in rural health.

Staff Present at Centre

1. Medical officer of Health-cum-lecturer/Assistant Professor
2. Lady medical officer
3. Medical social workers
4. Public health nurse
5. Health inspector
6. Health assistant (male)
7. Health educator
8. Technical assistant/technician
9. Store keeper-cum-record clerk
10. Peon
11. Van driver
12. Sweeper

Functions of RHTC

1. Curative services through outdoor and indoor (6 beds).
2. Child health services: Immunization, nutrition, growth monitoring, health education of mother and child health issues.
3. Maternal health care services: Antenatal natal and post-natal service, family welfare services including contraceptive distribution, education on health related issues of mother and children.
4. Education and training of medical students and interns on primary health care issues
5. Community health education
6. Participation in national health programmes
7. Survey and research activities
8. Organization of seminars
9. Training of health workers
10. Laboratory services like rapid detection kits for malaria parasites, routine and microscopic, hemoglobin estimation and blood and urine examination (UPT, sugar), etc.
11. Specialist services on periodical basis

Services Provided at RHTC

1. Medical care services through outdoor and indoor.
2. Referral services
3. Minor surgery
4. First aid/basic trauma management
5. Immunization of child and mother: At AWC, subcentre on MCHN day.
6. ANC check-up
7. Family planning and contraceptive distribution
8. Health education
9. Laboratory facility
10. Training and research activities, survey, etc.
11. Specialist services on periodical basis
12. School health programme

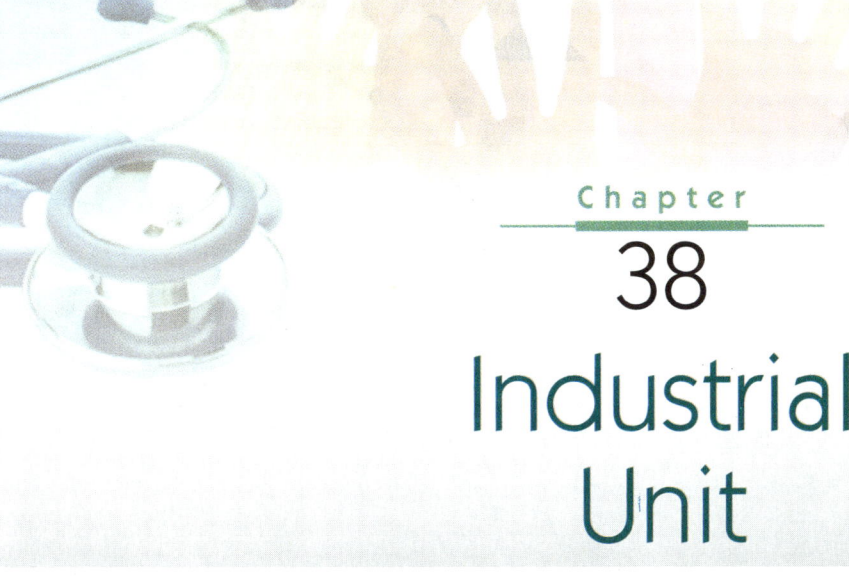

Competency		Suggested teaching	Suggested assessment
CM11.1	Enumerate and describe the presenting features of patients with occupational illness including agriculture	Lecture, small group discussion	Written/viva voce
CM11.2	Describe the role, benefits and functioning of the employees state insurance scheme	Lecture, small group discussion	Written/viva voce
CM11.3	Enumerate and describe specific occupational health hazards, their risk factors and preventive measures	Lecture, small group discussion	Written/viva voce
CM11.4	Describe the principles of ergonomics in health preservation	Small group discussion, lecture	Written/viva voce
CM11.5	Describe occupational disorders of health professionals and their prevention and management	Small group discussion, lecture	Written/viva voce

Brief Description of the Unit

Factory is an establishment employing 10 or more workers where power is used, and 20 or more workers where power is not used. The term 'worker' includes within its meaning contract labour employed in the manufacturing process.

What is Occupational Health? Describe Prevention and Control Strategies of Occupational Diseases.

According to *Joint Committee of WHO and ILO, 1950*, & occupational health aims at the promotion and maintenance of the highest degree of physical, mental and social well-being of workers in all occupations; the prevention amongst workers of departures from health caused by their working conditions; the protection of workers in their employment from risks resulting from factors adverse to health; placing and maintenance of the worker in an occupational environment adapted to his physiological and psychological equipment and to summarize: the adaptation of work to man and of each man to his job'.

Preventive Measures

1. Monitoring and evaluation of exposure
2. Engineering control measures
3. Preventing physical injuries
4. Minimizing the risk of heat illness
5. Personal protective equipment
6. Education and training
7. Health assessment

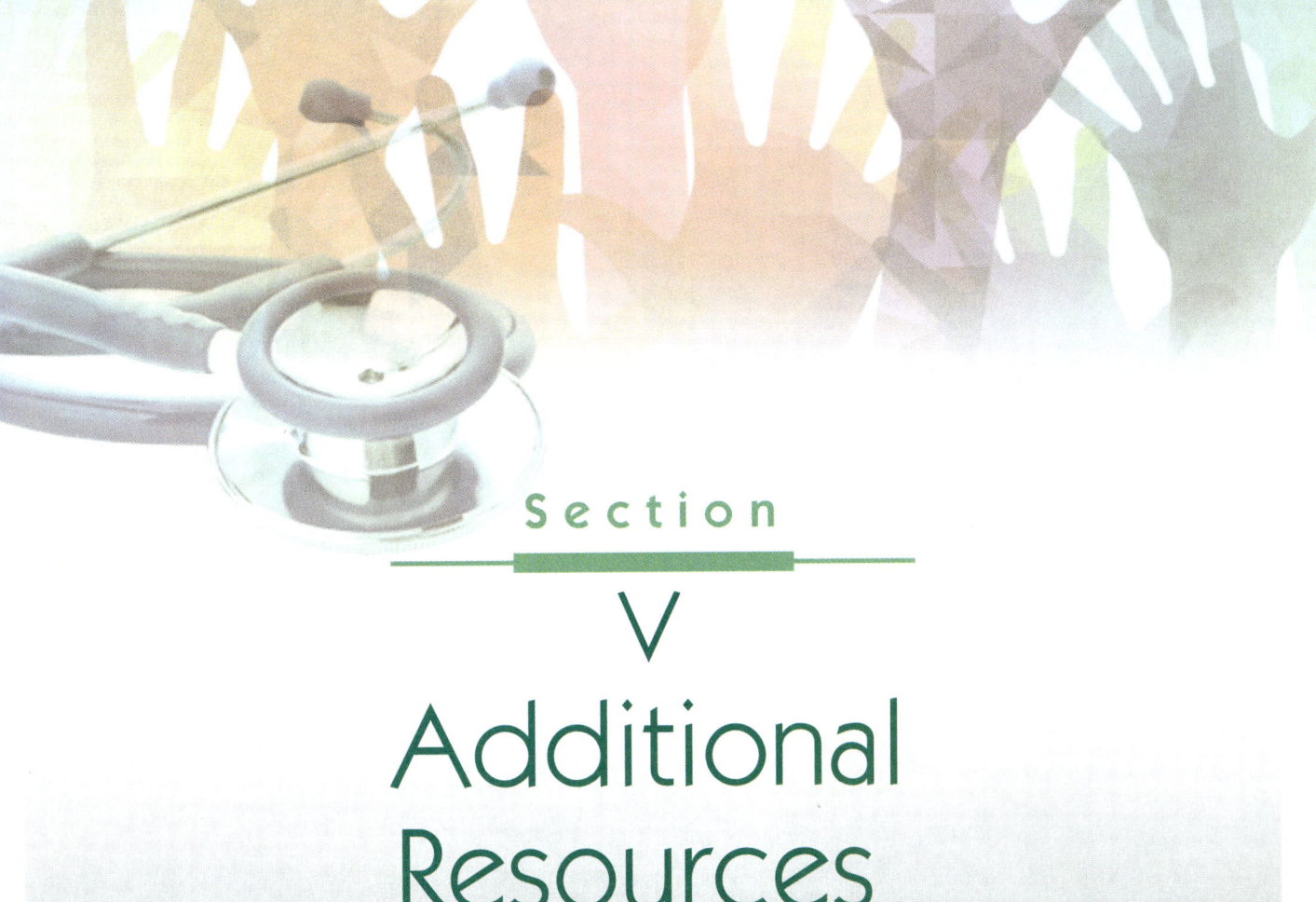

Section

V

Additional Resources

- ❖ Research Project
- ❖ Important Definitions

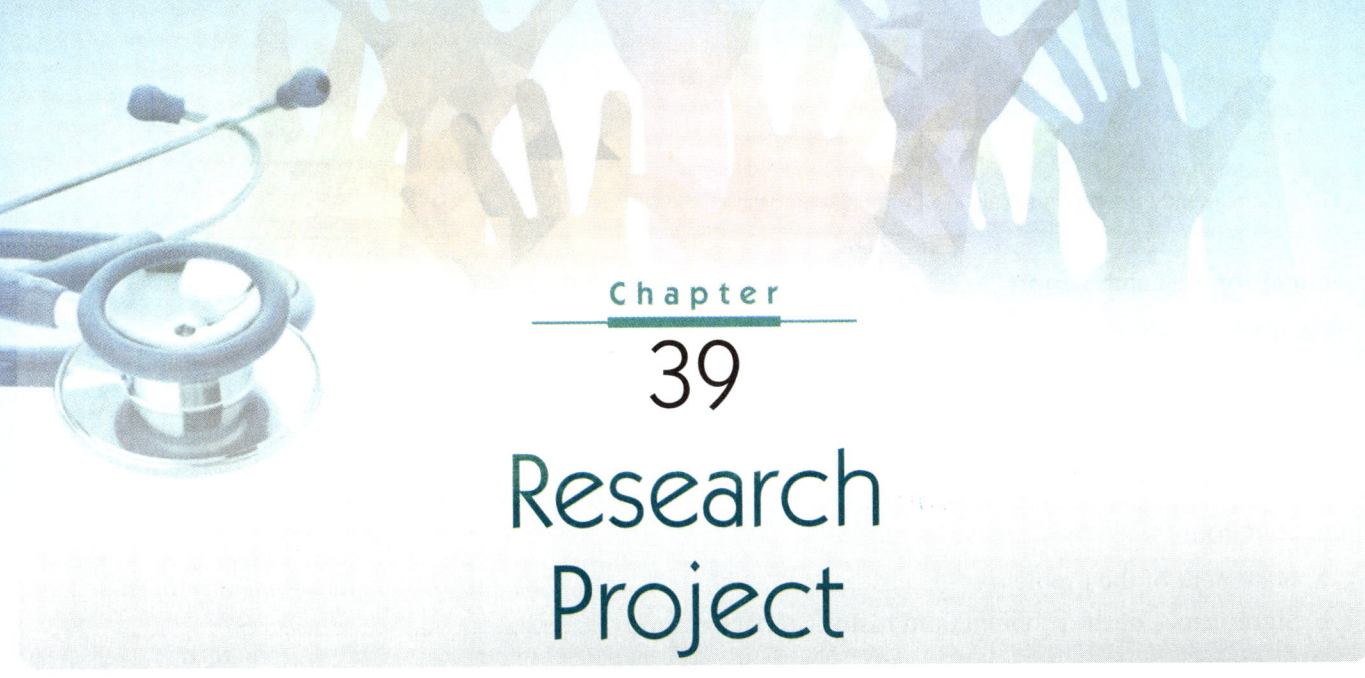

39
Research Project

The main objective of this chapter is to provide an opportunity to undergraduate medical students to familiarize themselves with research methodology and techniques by being associated for a short duration with their seniors on ongoing research program or by undertaking independent projects.

Examples of some research projects:

1. *A cross sectional study on assessing knowledge and skill of anganwadi workers in growth monitoring in an urban slum of central part of Karnataka.*

2. *Study of the impact of Menstrual practices on the health of adolescent girls and challenges faced in menstrual hygiene management at school.*

3. *A study on awareness about RNTCP and DOTS guidelines among health care professionals of tertiary care hospital.*

4. *Study of unmet needs for family planning among married women of reproductive age group attending on immunization clinic.*

5. *A study on medical and social audit of neonatal deaths, and status of their registration in a selected primary health centre.*

6. *Study of nutritional status and identification of associated risk factors in children below 5 years of age in a village.*

7. *Coverage evaluation of universal immunization program in PHC.*

8. *Migrant construction workers a morbidity study of marginalized population.*

9. *Cervical Cancer: How much women know, what they think and do? A hospital-based cross sectional study.*

10. *Misconceptions about diabetes mellitus in urban Pondicherry—barrier for effective prevention, control and treatment.*

11. *Evaluation of the revised national TB control programme (RNTCP).*

12. *Study on medical and social audit of neonatal deaths, and status of their registration in a selected primary health centre.*

13. *Osteoarthritis: Prevalence, health seeking behaviour and severity of disability; Cross sectional study*

14. *Study of feasibility and viability of mobile phone health care service provided to the rural population.*

15. *Awareness and perception regarding eye donation in rural Pondicherry.*

16. *An epidemiological study into risk factors of suicidal ideation and attempt among young and adult population.*

17. *A study to assess feasibility of Short Messaging Service in effectively delivering maternal and child healthcare messages in rural area of Tamil Nadu.*

Format for Research Report

Summary/Abstract: ....

Student Name and Guide: ....

Title: ....

Introduction

a. Statement of the problem ....

b. Significance of the problem (and historical background) ....

c. Purpose ....

d. Statement of hypothesis ....

e. Assumptions ....

f. Limitations ....

g. Definition of terms ....

h. Ethical considerations ....

i. Review of past literature ....

Methods

a. Description of research design and procedures used ....

b. Sources of data...

c. Sampling procedures ....

d. Methods and instruments of data gathering ....

e. Statistical treatment..

Results

a. Summary text with appropriate findings...

b. Tables ....

c. Figures ....

Conclusions

a. Restatement of the problem ....

b. Description of procedures ....

c. Major findings ....

d. Conclusions ....

e. Recommendations for further investigation ....

BIBLIOGRAPHY

1. Indian Council of Medical Research (ICMR): Short term studentship project and guidelines. Accessible from: http://14.139.60.56:84/Prepration_of_Proposal.aspx

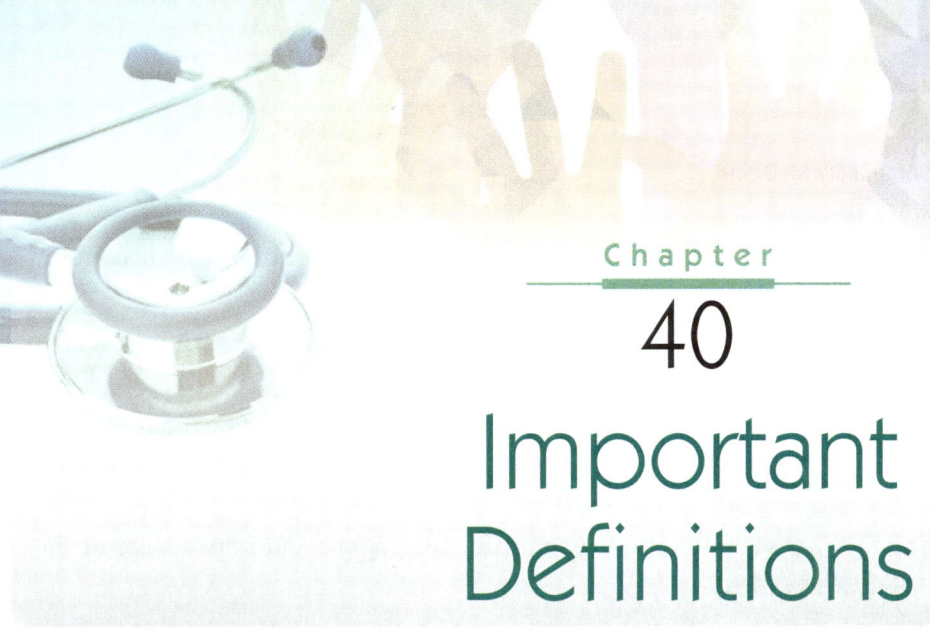

Important Definitions

Important Definitions

1. **Health:** A state of complete physical, mental and social well-being and not merely an absence of disease or infirmity, giving ability to lead a socially and economically productive life.

2. **Primary health care:** Essential health care based on practical, scientifically sound and socially acceptable methods and technology made universally accessible to individuals and families in the community through their full participation and at a cost that the community and the country can afford to maintain at every stage of their development in the spirit of self-determination.

3. **Disease control:** A process in which the disease agent is permitted to persist in the community at a level where it ceases to be a public health problem according to the tolerance of the local population. Examples: Measles, malaria.

4. **Disease elimination:** An interruption of transmission of disease. Example: Polio

5. **Disease eradication:** Termination of all transmission of infection by extermination of the infectious agent through surveillance and containment. Example: Smallpox.

6. **Monitoring:** The performance and analysis of routine measurements aimed at detecting changes in the environment or health status of population.

7. **Surveillance:** The continuous scrutiny of the factors that determine the occurrence and distribution of disease and other conditions of ill health. It is essential for effective control and prevention.

8. **Primordial prevention:** The prevention of the emergence or development of risk factors in countries or population groups in which they have not yet appeared.

9. **Primary prevention:** Action taken prior to the onset of disease, which removes the possibility that a disease will ever occur, signifying intervention in the pre-pathogenesis phase of a disease or health problems or other departure from health.

10. **Secondary prevention:** Action which halts the progress of a disease at its incipient stage and prevents complications. The specific interventions are early diagnosis and adequate treatment.

11. **Case:** A person in the population or study group identified as having the particular disease, health disorder or condition under investigation.

12. **Carrier:** An infected person or animal that harbours a specific infectious agent in the absence of discernible clinical disease and serves as a potential source of infection for others.

13. **Droplet nuclei:** Tiny particles (1–10 microns range) that represent the dried residue of droplets, which are implicated in the spread of airborne infection.

14. **Fomite-borne:** Inanimate articles or substances other than water or food contaminated by the infectious discharges from a patient and capable of harbouring and transferring the infectious agent to a healthy person.

15. **Incubation period:** The time interval between invasion by an infectious agent and appearance of the first sign or symptom of the disease in question.

16. **Communicable period:** Time during which an infectious agent may be transferred directly or indirectly from an infected person to another person, from an infected animal to man, or from an infected person to an animal, including arthropods.

17. **Herd immunity (community immunity):** A type of immunity that occurs when the vaccination of a portion of population (or herd) provides protection to unprotected individuals. It provides an immunological barrier to the spread of disease in the human herd.

18. **Vaccine:** An immuno-biological substance designed to produce specific protection against a given disease.

19. **Vaccine vial monitor (VVM):** A label containing a heat sensitive material, which is placed on a vaccine vial to register cumulative heat exposure over time.

20. **Isolation:** Separation for the period of communicability of infected persons or animals from others in such places and such conditions, as to prevent or limit the direct or indirect transmission of the infectious agent from those infected to those who are susceptible or who may spread the agent to others.

21. **Quarantine:** The limitation of freedom of movement of such well persons or domestic animals exposed to communicable disease for a period not longer than the longest usual incubation period of the disease, in such manner as to prevent effective contact with those not so exposed.

22. **Disinfection:** A process used to destroy pathogen and other types of microorganisms by thermal or chemical methods.

23. **Sterilization:** A process used to render a product free of all forms of viable microorganisms including bacterial spores.

24. **Screening:** The search for unrecognized disease or defect by means of rapidly applied tests, examinations or other procedures in apparently healthy individuals.

25. **Sensitivity:** The ability of a test to identify correctly all those who have the disease that is 'true positive.'

26. **Specificity:** The ability of a test to identify correctly those who do not have the disease that is "true negative".

27. **Lead time:** The interval between the point a condition is detected through screening and the time it would normally have been detected due to appearance and reporting of signs and symptoms.

28. **Lag time:** Time interval between two closely related events to like between stimulus and response.

29. **Impairment:** Any loss or any abnormality of psychological or anatomical structure or function. Example: Loss of foot, defective vision, etc.

30. **Disability:** Any restriction or lack of ability to perform an activity in the manner or within the range considered normal for a human being. Example: Inability to walk.

31. **Handicap:** A disadvantage for a given individual, resulting from impairment or a disability that limits or prevents the fulfilment of a role that is normal (depending on age, sex, and social and cultural factors) for that individual. Example: Loss of job.

32. **Epidemiology:** The study of the distribution and determinants of health-related states or events in specified populations, and the application of this study to the control of health problems.

33. **Incidence:** The number of new cases occurring in a defined population during a specified period of time.

34. **Prevalence:** The total number of all individuals who have an attribute or a disease at a particular time (or during a particular period) divided by the population at risk having the attribute or disease at this point in time or midway through the period.

35. **Secondary attack rate:** The number of exposed persons developing the disease within the range of the incubation period following exposure to a primary case.

36. **Epidemic:** The "unusual" occurrence in a community or region of disease, specific health related behaviour or other health related events clearly in excess of "expected occurrence".

37. **Outbreak:** A small usually localised epidemic in the interest of minimizing public alarm, unless the number of cases is indeed very large.

38. **Endemic:** The constant presence of a disease or infectious agent within a given geographic area or population group, without importation from outside. Example: Japanese encephalitis in selected districts in India.

39. **Sporadic:** The cases occurring irregularly, haphazardly from time to time, and generally infrequently. Example: Herpes zoster, meningococcal meningitis.

40. **Pandemic:** An epidemic usually affecting a large proportion of the population, occurring over a wide geographic area such as a section of a nation, the entire nation, a continent or the world. Examples: H1N1 influenza (2009), COVID-19(2020).

41. **Zoonosis:** An infection or infectious disease transmissible under natural conditions from vertebrate animals to man. Examples: Rabies, plague, anthrax, brucellosis, bovine TB, etc.

Index